DR. COLBERT'S

HORMONE HEALTH ZONE

DON COLBERT, MD

SILOAM

Most CHARISMA HOUSE BOOK GROUP products are available at special quantity discounts for bulk purchase for sales promotions, premiums, fund-raising, and educational needs. For details, write Charisma House Book Group, 600 Rinehart Road, Lake Mary, Florida 32746, or telephone (407) 333-0600.

DR. COLBERT'S HORMONE HEALTH ZONE by Don Colbert, MD
Published by Siloam
Charisma Media/Charisma House Book Group
600 Rinehart Road
Lake Mary, Florida 32746
www.charismahouse.com

All Scripture quotations are taken from the New King James Version®. Copyright © 1982 by Thomas Nelson. Used by permission. All rights reserved.

Illustrations by Abraham Mast

Visit the author's website at www.drcolbert.com or hormonehealthbook.com.

Library of Congress Cataloging-in-Publication Data

Names: Colbert, Don, author.
Title: Dr. Colbert's hormone health zone / Don Colbert.
Description: Lake Mary, Florida : Siloam, [2019]
Identifiers: LCCN 2018054892 (print) | LCCN 2018056420 (ebook) | ISBN 9781629995748 (e-book) | ISBN 9781629995731 (hardback) | ISBN 9781629995748 (ebook)
Subjects: LCSH: Hormone therapy--Popular works. | Rejuvenation. | Women--Health and hygiene. | Men--Health and hygiene. | Self-care, Health--Popular works. | BISAC: HEALTH & FITNESS / Naturopathy. | HEALTH & FITNESS / Women's Health. | HEALTH & FITNESS / Men's Health. | HEALTH & FITNESS / Alternative Therapies.
Classification: LCC RM286 (ebook) | LCC RM286 .C65 2019 (print) | DDC 615.3/6--dc23
LC record available at https://lccn.loc.gov/2018054892

This book contains the opinions and ideas of its author. It is solely for informational and educational purposes and should not be regarded as a substitute

Author's note: For years, I have told couples not to get divorced until they both get their hormones checked, balanced, and optimized. Every marriage counselor, family counselor, psychologist, and pastor should know this! I have seen hundreds of marriages restored after they both got their testosterone levels back on track. This is obviously not all about sex; this is about life, marriage, family, fun, health, and being all that we were meant to be. How can we bring glory and honor to God when our lives are falling apart? Of course hormone levels are not the answer to everything, but they do play an important part in every area of life, especially your marriage.

This publication is translated in Spanish under the title *La zona de salud hormonal*, copyright © 2019 by Don Colbert, MD, published by Casa Creación, a Charisma Media company. All rights reserved.

19 20 21 22 23 — 8 7 6 5 4
Printed in the United States of America

To all the millions of patients who have been told that their symptoms including fatigue, cold hands, cold feet, brain fog, lethargy, depressed mood, irritability, and more were due to aging or stress or depression. You were probably prescribed an antidepressant and other meds and told with a pat on the back that it's a normal part of aging and to expect more troublesome symptoms. Well, you probably need your hormones optimized or brought to the level of a twenty-five-year-old. When that happens, most of these symptoms are relieved.

CONTENTS

HOW HEALTHY DO YOU WANT TO BE?

I**T ISN'T VERY** often, at least in the medical community, that you can look at a very real need, such as a debilitating sickness or decade-long symptoms, and say, "We now have an answer for that." The word that best describes this feeling is *hope*. Maybe *excitement* as well!

This book contains answers to so many symptoms, diseases, sicknesses, ailments, troubles, and problems that I cannot list them all! The prospects for better health and an improved future have never been brighter! The question really is, How healthy do you want to be?

We all naturally want to be as healthy as possible. After all, our health is our greatest commodity. It is what gives us the opportunity to pursue our goals, reach our dreams, and enjoy life to the fullest.

Sadly many of us have limits. Some we impose on ourselves; others are imposed on us. As a result, we have "health caps" that seem insurmountable. "Well, that's what happens when you turn thirty, forty, fifty, or sixty," we are told. Whatever the age, there is a long list of ailments that are supposedly normal to have. But I don't want them; do you?

What if we could exchange all the "normal," negative symptoms for such things as:

- increased metabolism
- better sleep
- more energy
- greater focus
- weight loss
- improved stamina
- lower cholesterol

- for women, getting your curves back
- for men, no erectile dysfunction
- thick hair
- wrinkle-free skin
- dementia protection
- Alzheimer's protection
- Parkinson's protection
- warm hands and warm feet
- hope and zest for life

"Sign me up for those symptoms," people would gladly say. Thankfully we can usually do just that when we *optimize* our hormone levels. We have been told for years that our hormones need to be balanced, but as we will discuss more in the book, that is not a complete picture.

Think of it this way: imagine you have been training to run a local 5K race, and when you show up to get your jersey, you are given the choice of carrying a one hundred–pound rock, a fifty-pound rock, or no rock at all.

If your hormones are out of whack, it's like you've got the one hundred–pound rock to deal with. And if your hormones are balanced, then you get the much lighter, fifty-pound rock to tote around. That's better, you think, but what about the zero-pound option? That's when your hormones are beyond balanced; they're *optimized*, which is what this book is about.

You can also think of it as a grade. Scoring a D- grade is still technically passing, but barely...and that is similar to when someone is barely in the normal range for hormones. An average grade of C is similar to patients who have their hormones balanced and at mid-range. An A grade, however, is when your hormones have reached optimized levels.

That is the way it is with hormones. Even when they are balanced, we are still typically running at a deficit. Usually we're dealing with some symptoms, disease is knocking at the door, and life is hard going. Some may claim they are happy with balanced hormone levels, but given a chance to choose between balanced and optimized, I'm guessing they would opt for optimized hormones.

For decades I have helped patients balance their hormones, and only rarely did they say, "I feel great!" Sure, they feel better than they did, but they usually don't feel great. Yes, they traded a one hundred–pound rock for a fifty-pound rock or the D grade for a C grade. It's lighter, and that makes life better, but who wants to just cope with life? To truly feel great is to run free, to be healthy and whole, and to enjoy life. That is how our bodies were intended to run.

So if you want to move from feeling fair or better to feeling great, to close the door on numerous diseases, to get back to looking and feeling as you did when you were younger, and to regain your competitive edge, then *optimizing your hormones* is the way to go. It is a delightful journey and one that you will probably enjoy for the rest of your life!

IT'S TIME TO GET IN THE ZONE

N UMEROUS EPIDEMICS ARE sweeping the United States. Here are just a few:

- Obesity: nearly two in five (39.8 percent) of us are now obese.[1]
- Type 2 diabetes and prediabetes: approximately one in ten of us is diabetic, and one in three has prediabetes.[2]
- Heart disease: one in four deaths is from heart disease.[3]
- Alzheimer's: in 2013 it's estimated that Alzheimer's affected five million Americans; experts anticipate this to almost triple by 2050.[4]

As adults age, their quality of life slowly deteriorates, and they become more fatigued, more apathetic, more stressed, and eventually depressed. They gain weight, and their doctor usually starts prescribing more and more medications, including statin drugs to lower cholesterol, antidepressants to treat depression, antihypertensive medications for high blood pressure, diabetic medication for type 2 diabetes and prediabetes, and sleeping pills for insomnia. But are the medications prescribed to treat disease and symptoms really getting to the root of the problem?

IT'S A FACT

Did you know in this country adverse drug reactions are now the fourth-leading cause of death? That puts them ahead of diabetes, pulmonary disease, AIDS, pneumonia, automobile deaths, and accidents.[5] Think about that before your doctor writes another prescription.

The root cause of many diseases and ailments associated with aging—obesity, prediabetes, type 2 diabetes, fatigue, depression, stress overload, heart disease, high cholesterol, and hypertension—is usually suboptimal hormone levels, including sex hormones, thyroid hormones, and adrenal hormones.

Yes, diet and nutrition are important, but optimizing your hormones is absolutely the key to feeling great, losing weight, and having energy, vitality, passion, stamina, and strength. The good news is that in this book I'm going to tell you how to do just that. You don't want just to survive; you want to thrive! What is more, when you optimize your hormones, you become resistant to most of the diseases associated with aging!

Now let's look at a few hormones and their benefits.

BENEFITS OF OPTIMIZING TESTOSTERONE LEVELS FOR BOTH MEN AND WOMEN

- Helps you lose weight and build muscle. And the more muscle you have, the higher your metabolic rate and the more calories you burn at rest. This helps prevent prediabetes and type 2 diabetes, and along with a proper diet, it may even reverse type 2 diabetes entirely.

- Increases energy, which elevates your mood, and that in turn usually helps improve or overcome depression. After all, optimal energy and good mood are essential to compete and win in a competitive world.

- Protects your brain, improves memory, and prevents dementia. It prevents shrinkages of the brain, improves blood flow in the brain, and helps repair neurons in the brain.

- Builds strong bones.

- Protects your heart by increasing nitric oxide, which improves blood flow in the coronary arteries.

Testosterone strengthens the heart muscle, which helps maintain strong heart contractions.

- Provides one of the best antidepressants by increasing the neurotransmitters, including norepinephrine, serotonin, and dopamine.[6]
- Decreases inflammation in your body, which helps reduce chronic pain and pain from arthritis and fibromyalgia.
- Prevents feebleness and frailty, which I believe is the best insurance to keep you out of the nursing home as you age. (That is why I have optimized my mother's testosterone levels, which I'll share more about later.)

Benefits of Optimizing Thyroid Levels With Active Thyroid*

- Usually increases your energy better than most other hormones or supplements I have seen.
- Usually helps you lose weight by increasing the metabolic rate.
- Improves and may correct depression by elevating your mood.
- Helps improve infertility and heavy menstrual bleeding.
- Improves muscle aches and pains and usually improves fibromyalgia.
- Usually helps stop hair loss, especially when combined with bioidentical micronized progesterone.
- Usually improves memory.
- Often improves or corrects constipation.
- Commonly lowers cholesterol significantly and often helps prevent plaque buildup in the arteries.
- Heats the body up and resolves the cold hands and cold feet commonly seen with low or suboptimal thyroid.

---

* 99 percent of prescriptions use inactive thyroid in the form of Synthroid or levothyroxine.

Optimizing these hormones, along with bioidentical estradiol, progesterone, and adrenal hormones, is vital in preventing diseases associated with aging. In *Dr. Colbert's Hormone Health Zone*, I will teach you how to enter and stay "in the zone," which will prevent and/or treat countless diseases.

I have had patients in their fifties, sixties, seventies, eighties, and early nineties who are disease-free and who have tremendous energy, passion, and vitality. They are living in the hormone health zone.

Being in the hormone health zone is not only balancing your hormones but also optimizing them so that your hormones are at the level of a healthy twenty-five-year-old man or woman. You then usually start to feel like a twenty-five-year-old yourself! Patients who live in the hormone health zone are the healthiest, most disease-resistant patients that I encounter and are busy doing what they enjoy in life. They are doers, not sitting and resting and doing nothing.

For almost three decades I balanced hormones with bioidentical hormones, but over the past few years I have shifted to optimizing hormones with amazing results. We are talking about preventing and reversing diseases in the lives of countless patients. So impressive are the results that I call the hormone health zone the eighth pillar of health.

Personally, I have been living in the hormone health zone for the past few years and have more energy, strength, and vitality than I had at twenty years of age. I regret not finding out about this earlier because I could have done so much more if I had lived more of my life in the hormone health zone.

Now you have the opportunity to live in the hormone health zone. Slam the door on most diseases associated with aging, and start to feel like a twenty-five-year-old again by getting in the zone!

PART I
MAKING SENSE OF HORMONES

PART 1 IS an effort to make sense of the often confusing role of hormones in our lives and our health. It clarifies the confusion, shows what the symptoms mean, and provides answers. This explains just what happened to our hormones.

CHAPTER 1

HORMONES . . . AND THE LIFE YOU WANT

B ILL HAD BEEN a patient of mine for several years. At age eighty he was constantly tired, had chronic back pain and arthritis, could hardly get out of bed, couldn't sleep well at night, and had an enlarged prostate. As I worked to manage his health problems, which also included some brain fog, mild depression, and increasingly cold hands and cold feet, I balanced his hormones. I was careful not to push his testosterone hormone levels too high.

The problem was that his long list of symptoms never seemed to go away. All he wanted to do was sit around the house, read the paper, and watch the news. Basically he felt like doing nothing. He was turning into a grumpy, irritable old man!

"That's what happens when you are eighty," he joked, but I knew he wanted more out of life. So did I—and not only for him but for myself when I reached that age.

Bill's testosterone levels hovered around 500 ng/dL, and with the range for men being 348–1197 ng/dL at that time, Bill was pretty middle-of-the-road. His hormones were balanced, and we had worked to get them there. Without the work we had done, his hormone numbers would have been much lower.

One day Bill flew across the country to visit a fellow eighty-year-old friend in California. Besides being the same age, not much was similar. His friend still had broad shoulders and a narrow waist, and he was active. He played tennis or golf every other day, had tremendous energy, went on vacations, and was having fun. In fact, he had so much energy that he was volunteering with a charity to raise money for a cause he believed in.

"What are you doing that I'm not?" Bill demanded soon after he arrived.

His friend explained, "I keep my hormones at the level of a twenty-year-old."

"What? My hormones are balanced," Bill pressed. "They are within range, as they should be."

"They might be balanced, but they are balanced at the level you would expect of a sixty-, seventy-, or eighty-year-old guy, right?" his friend teased.

Intrigued, Bill asked, "So what exactly do you do to get your hormone levels to those of a twenty-year-old?"

"The answer is hormone injections. I've been doing it for a few years now, and I feel great," Bill's friend stated emphatically.

Bill was sick and tired of his symptoms, and since he was in town for several weeks, he made an appointment to see his friend's local doctor. After the blood tests, they set the goal to raise his testosterone and thyroid levels to those of a twenty-year-old.

Anxious to change his life, Bill learned to give himself the shots, which turned out to be a lot less painful and far easier than he expected. His testosterone levels went up to around 950 ng/dL, and within a few months all his symptoms began to go away.

First to leave were his brain fog and depression, and he had greater stamina and focus. Next went the back pain and arthritis. He had more energy and didn't need so many naps throughout the day. He began to exercise more, which included walking, biking, and core-strengthening exercises. Within nine months he was a different man.

When he came to see me, he told me point-blank, "I want to keep my hormones at the level of a twenty-year-old."

"What do you mean?" I asked. "You are almost eighty-one."

He explained what he had been doing since his last checkup. The more we talked, the more I found myself agreeing with him. And why not? Why just balance your hormones when you can optimize them?

But is it healthy? Will it hurt him? Are there negative side effects that could outweigh the good side effects? I checked his PSA (prostate-specific antigen) numbers, and they were fine. In fact, his urinary frequency had even improved.

And so began my transition from balancing hormones to optimizing them.

Getting the Most Out of Life

It has been several years since that discussion with Bill. In his own independent-thinking ways, he pushed me to reconsider what I was taught and my subsequent treatment of patients.

I began attending advanced hormone training by some of the top antiaging experts, gynecologists, and hormone doctors in the world. It took a lot of time, effort, and money to learn how to detect suboptimal hormone levels, treat the various hormones in the best possible way, and optimize hormone levels to the point where patients are able to regain their health.

And the difference in my patients' lives? It has been amazing! I could tell stories for hours, such as:

- stories of young women who could not get pregnant, much less carry their babies to term, who now have one or more children of their own

- stories of men who were able to fix the real issue and no longer suffer from the symptoms of erectile dysfunction

- stories of women who were able to get completely off their antidepressant medications

- stories of aging men who were able to rebuild muscle and actually stop the gradual slide of muscle loss

- stories of women who escaped the nightmare of migraines, weight gain, irritability, anxiety, or PMS

- stories of men and women who stopped cold the onset of memory-related diseases

- stories of men and women who no longer suffer from high blood pressure, insomnia, high cholesterol, type 2 diabetes, fibromyalgia, chronic fatigue, or chronic pain

- stories of elderly men and women who can continue to live their lives as they choose, and that includes not being admitted into a nursing home

Trust me when I say the stories are endless, all because we were able to optimize hormone levels.

FROM BALANCING TO OPTIMIZING

Finding what is best for patients also must include what is healthy for them. Though that should go without saying, I work very diligently to test, recheck, and watch lab tests and hormone levels so that the patients' improved lives stay that way. Also included are diet, exercise, nutritional supplementation, and lifestyle habits, but at the center of the transformation in these people's lives is the simple fact that we optimize their hormones.

I have been practicing medicine now for thirty-five years and bioidentical hormone replacement therapy for more than twenty-five of those years. During that time I have found that truly helping patients get to the root cause of their issues takes longer than a five-to-ten-minute office visit. It also requires more than a simple "take this pill and come back in six months" prescription.

IT'S A FACT

Close to 70 percent of Americans are on one medication; more than 50 percent are on two.[1]

Years ago I had one of the busiest doctor's offices in the state of Florida, but today I only see about eight people a day. Yes, it limits my income, but I refuse to compromise the health care my patients truly need. They need a plan, one that includes lifestyle, dietary, hormonal, and nutritional elements so they can actually get better.

I will say that when they come through the office door, I know almost everything medical about them. They fill out countless history forms and questionnaires and send me all their previous reports before they come in. I know every complaint, blood test, past surgery, sleep issue, exercise habit, food they eat, personal issue, vital sign, and much more.

During our hour-long office visit all the pieces come together, enabling us to focus like a laser on creating a plan to meet their needs and address their very real symptoms. They come back several months later, and we adjust the details that need to be adjusted. Usually within three to six months the patient is a completely transformed person!

When the symptoms disappear, the diseases usually leave or improve, and joy, life, excitement, health, and vigor return! That is the reason why I do what I do!

Sadly the answer most patients get from their primary care doctors regarding their symptoms that never seem to improve is another medication. That either makes the situation worse or creates a whole new list of negative side effects.

Believe it or not, most people who have brain fog, sluggishness, depression, weight gain, insomnia, slow metabolism, erectile dysfunction, cold hands, memory issues, muscle loss, and so on are not going to find the answers they need by taking a medication.

And when the real reason for the symptom is not addressed, things usually only get worse. That in turn opens the door to other diseases and other medications to treat the new symptoms, and the cycle continues downward for the patient.

There is a much, much better way. Optimizing hormones is a big part of that answer.

TexAS
Lake mary

CHAPTER 2

WHY ALL THE HORMONE CONFUSION?

TRISHA HAD BEEN misdiagnosed. I could tell that within a few minutes of meeting her.

"My doctor has me taking antidepressant medication, and he wants to put me on some other drug as well. I just don't want to take all these medications, but I have to do something about feeling like a slug. I'm bone-tired, and with brain fog I feel as if I can hardly think. Going to sleep at night is getting harder and harder. All combined, it's messing with my job performance."

She was only thirty-nine years old, had three young children, and worked in an accounting office. She was not the only breadwinner in the family, but she could not afford to lose her job.

"What's more, I can't seem to lose weight as easily as I used to. I would simply cut out desserts and work out at the gym a little harder, but now it makes no difference. I've stopped eating sweets entirely, but the extra fifteen pounds just won't leave my belly."

The more we talked, the more it was obvious. Her hormones were out of balance, and the imbalance was only going to get worse if we didn't do something about it right away.

We ran several blood tests, which confirmed it. Her hormone numbers, especially her thyroid and testosterone, were at the lower end of the medical industry's acceptable range. Had her doctor run the same tests, he probably would not have done anything about it. After all, she was still "in range."

I explained how her symptoms matched her hormone levels. I also added that hormones can easily be messed up by stress, chemicals, and aging.

"I hate aging!" she exclaimed.

"Don't we all," I laughed.

"As for stress, I've got plenty of that with the kids, my boss, the daily commute, my in-laws, and even our neighbors. I don't know what it is, but stress seems to be a constant in our lives."

She was, though she didn't know it, incredibly normal. We have more stressors today than we did just one generation ago.

"I don't know about the chemicals, but we try to eat healthily," she added. "And we both go to the gym regularly."

"The food and exercise we will talk about later," I explained. "First up are your hormones. We need to optimize those. That in turn will probably address the symptoms you have, including tiredness, trying to lose weight, insomnia, lack of energy, and brain fog."

We came up with a plan, and she was eager to get started. We talked briefly about hormones, how bioidentical hormones are natural and safe, and how optimizing hormone levels can actually counter many of our age-related symptoms and illnesses.

Within a few weeks of starting the hormone replacement therapy, she was feeling much improved. At her six-week checkup she was ecstatic.

"I feel incredible," she chimed. "I really do. My energy levels are up, I feel 'on' all day long, and I have no brain fog whatsoever." Her hormone numbers were indeed better. They were just past the middle of the road, on their way up toward the upper range of normal.

Three months later her numbers were running near the top of the range in both thyroid and testosterone levels. The dose was good, and the plan was working. She had already lost five pounds, she was sleeping great, and her mood was very cheerful.

Then her doctor had her stop in to discuss the second medication he wanted her to take. Within seconds she was telling him how good she was feeling, what she was doing, and how she probably didn't need the new medication or the antidepressant any longer.

That was when he dropped it on her. "You want to get cancer?" he asked.

"Well, no," she stammered.

"I would not take any hormone therapy. It causes breast cancer and blood clots and raises your blood pressure. All of this has been well documented," he stated.

She didn't know how to reply.

An hour later she called my office to see if she could set up a quick appointment. I happened to have a window of time the next morning, and she came in crying.

"I feel so good, I don't want to stop," she said, sniffling, "but I obviously don't want to get cancer. What do I do?"

What would you do?

Thankfully her story ends well. I showed her the medical studies that refuted the common fears of many doctors, and she decided to continue with the hormones. She is doing great today, has a clean bill of health (by her primary care doctor), and continues to take her hormone replacement therapy.

I have had other patients who chose to follow their doctors' or endocrinologists' warnings. Within a few months of stopping the hormone replacement therapy, their symptoms were back, and they felt horrible again. The only option at that point was taking whatever medications the doctor recommended.

You are the one who decides what your health will be.

As for hormones, there is indeed a lot of confusion on the subject. That should not be the case. I will do my best to highlight some of the most common points of confusion. You can then make your decision based on facts.

Eight Causes of Hormone Confusion

With all the negative symptoms, epidemics, sicknesses, and diseases that can successfully be treated with hormone therapy, why is there so much confusion on the subject?

You would think we would be past all that and into the widespread use of hormone therapy to treat patients, save lives, prevent disease, drive down health care costs, and improve the quality of life across the board and around the globe. In time it will happen, but for now we have to work on overcoming all the confusion.

1. "It's a woman thing."

Hormones have typically been seen as a "woman" issue, but not anymore. Hormone replacement therapy is needed by men as much as it is needed by women. The only reason women potentially require more hormone replacement therapy is that they have one extra hormone needing replacement (progesterone) that men don't need to replace, but I would not be surprised if the demand for hormone replacement therapy among men surpasses that of women in the next ten years.

Here is a reality check that will strike a little fear into a lot of men: if you are not working on keeping yourself in shape and are getting belly fat, especially if you are growing a pair of "man boobs," your testosterone levels are probably getting low, and your estrogen levels are getting too high! You had better work on that pronto.

Hormones are not a woman thing; hormones are a human thing, and both men and women need to pay attention to their hormone levels.

2. "All hormones are created equal."

Regardless of what people might say or wish to believe, not all hormones are created equal. A synthetic or nonbioidentical hormone is not the same as a bioidentical hormone. One is a good match and works well with your body at the cellular level, and the other does not.

Synthetic, or nonbioidentical, hormones can still bind to hormone receptors, but the message is usually not exactly like the messages produced by the body's hormones. This different chemical structure results in less-effective treatment of symptoms. The bioidentical hormones, however, have the same chemical composition as hormones produced in the body and therefore can perform all the functions required of the hormones.

One very common nonbioidentical hormone is Premarin, which is made of a mix of estrone (the last type of estrogen a woman wants in her body, often called "old lady estrogen") and horse estrogen from the urine of pregnant mares. Approximately half of the estrogens in Premarin are the horse estrogens equilin and equilenin. The results are not that good, and the side effects are often worse.

IT'S A FACT

The synthetic T4 thyroid medication called Synthroid has been the most prescribed drug in America for years, with millions of prescriptions written each year![1]

What is more, Premarin is taken in pill form. That is the worst way to deliver estrogen into the body because it goes into the gut, then the liver, and that usually creates other adverse reactions in your body, such as elevated blood pressure, elevated liver enzymes, weight gain, elevated triglycerides, and an increased risk of gallstones.

Nonbioidentical and synthetic hormones can be patented, which means big money to pharmaceutical companies, while natural bioidentical hormones cannot be patented. Whether that is a driving force behind the number of prescriptions is a separate debate. What concerns me as a doctor is how often synthetic hormones are prescribed, along with all the negative side effects, when bioidentical hormones are readily available and have far fewer side effects.

Simply stated, hormones are far from equal.

3. "Hormone therapy causes breast cancer."

In addition to supposedly causing breast cancer, hormone therapy is claimed to also cause high blood pressure, heart attacks, and blood clots. Obviously nobody wants that, but is it true? Not for bioidentical hormones because they actually provide protection from heart disease and do not increase the risk of blood clots, Alzheimer's, breast cancer, or other chronic illnesses.[2]

I cannot say the same for synthetic and nonbioidentical hormones. More than fifteen different studies found that synthetic progesterone, progestin, significantly increases breast cell growth.[3] Recently eleven different studies found that bioidentical progesterone does not cause estrogen-stimulated breast cell proliferation, which is part of the breast cancer growth process.[4] I have seen the results of synthetic and nonbioidentical hormones in my patients. They include such things as uncontrolled weight gain, depression, increased risk for breast cancer, bad cholesterol (LDL) rising and good cholesterol (HDL) lowering, and memory loss, not to mention sex drive being completely destroyed. So the correct question would seem to be whether or not *synthetic* hormones cause diseases. I believe they do.

I will add that I'm frequently asked if bioidentical hormones are safe even if someone already has cancer. If someone has or has had breast, uterine, or ovarian cancer, that person should avoid bioidentical estrogen. I do not recommend bioidentical estrogen for patients with breast, uterine, or ovarian cancer. Additionally someone who currently has other types of cancer needs to be extra cautious with bioidentical hormone therapy.

4. "My doctor says it's something else."

We have symptoms, and we go to the doctor. Whatever ails us, from insomnia to migraines to brain fog to hot flashes to diabetes to erectile dysfunction to weight gain, doctors do their best to treat us. The wrong diagnosis will clearly lead to the wrong treatment. In time the real issue, which has never been addressed, will usually simply be worse than it was, and other symptoms (usually directly related to the medicines we are given) will show up, which then need their own set of countering medicines.

IT'S A FACT

Do you suffer from fatigue, depression, anxiety, aches, pains, or insomnia? The usual prescription is for antidepressants, sleeping pills, and pain medication...but your hormones are probably suboptimal. The medication may make things worse.

Take depression, for example. If patients say they are tired, stressed, depressed, anxious, or something common like that, an antidepressant is quickly prescribed. That is why antidepressants, including for teens and preteens, constantly rank as one of the top prescriptions given out in the United States.[5] The known side effects of antidepressants include such things as insomnia, nausea, anxiety, restlessness, dizziness, decreased sex drive, sweating, weight gain, dry mouth, tremors, fatigue, diarrhea, constipation, and headaches.[6] This creates a vicious cycle because many of these symptoms, such as insomnia, anxiety, or decreased sex drive, usually constitute prescribing another medication.

I treat patients with depression all the time—especially women—and more than ninety times out of one hundred, when we balance and optimize their hormones, their depression goes away. Not only that, but they usually get their energy back, they sleep well, their mood is improved, and they don't experience that long list of unpleasant side effects. If you battle depression, are you interested in an effective way to treat it without negative side effects such as those listed above? Who wouldn't be!

Drugs that lower your cholesterol are also commonly prescribed. Did you know cholesterol-lowering drugs also lower your testosterone level, and depression, weight gain, lower sex drive, less energy, brain fog, muscle loss, hair loss, and poor memory often follow decreased testosterone levels? No thanks!

At the point of diagnosis, when doctors only have ten to fifteen minutes to talk with you, it is understandable that a quick fix would be prescribed. But just because they give it to you does not mean you need to take it. Get a second or third opinion.

5. "My doctor says my hormones are in range."

One fact that all people, doctors and patients alike, have to look at is the numbers associated with their hormone levels. You get your blood work done to check your hormone levels, but the different lab companies that run the blood tests, such as LabCorp or Quest Diagnostics, have differing ranges for normal, and those usually change and may be lowered every few years. Also, the numbers are measured in different ways: ng/dL (nanograms per deciliter), pg/mL (picograms per milliliter), and µIU/mL (micro-international units per milliliter) to name a few. That alone can be confusing.

But without question the hardest part for anyone to understand is the incredibly wide range for each of your hormones. Take testosterone, for example. I have seen many men (such as Bill in the first chapter) who had low testosterone levels, but the range when I first treated him was 348–1197 ng/dL.

The "normal" range for testosterone is moving lower and lower as the population gets fatter and fatter. Only a few years ago it was 348–1197 ng/dL; now it has been lowered to 264–916 ng/dL. A male with testosterone levels around 300 ng/dL is most likely going to be battling obesity, erectile dysfunction, lethargy, lack of muscle, high cholesterol, plaque in his arteries, brain fog, type 2 diabetes or pre-diabetes, and a host of other ailments. Yet he is in the normal range! How can he and a man who suffers none of these symptoms and has a testosterone level around 900 ng/dL both be considered in the normal range? It makes no sense.

The same issue affects both men and women with the free T3 (thyroid) hormone. The suggested range is 2.0–4.4 pg/mL, but someone with free T3 numbers around 2.0 is most likely going to feel terrible, have trouble losing weight, experience fatigue, have cold hands and cold feet, battle depression and irritability, suffer hair loss, and even lose the hair on their outer eyebrows. How can that be normal?

At the end of the day whatever the numbers are, they are *your* numbers. If you have symptoms because your numbers are low, then you may need bioidentical hormone replacement therapy to bring those numbers up. And if you want to optimize your numbers and get all the benefits that go with it, then therapy is certainly needed.

Unsure of what to do? Trust your body and your symptoms more than you trust the ranges, and then take action.

6. "My doctor doesn't test for that."

It would seem simple enough. You go to your doctor, describe your symptoms, get blood work to prove you right or wrong, and take action accordingly. It does seem simple.

But a typical doctor usually has no time to dig deep enough to find the core issue that ails you. He checks your complete blood count (CBC) to see if you are anemic, a chemistry panel to see if your electrolytes are normal and your liver and kidney are functioning well, and a lipid panel to see how cholesterol is doing. (About one-third of Americans have high cholesterol.[7]) Maybe if you mention hormones, they will recommend the thyroid-stimulating hormone (TSH) thyroid screen. Almost always the numbers are in range, so no action is needed.

Unbeknownst to most people, doctors included, the TSH test is most accurate at seeing if your brain and pituitary have sufficient levels of thyroid hormone. It's not accurate for seeing thyroid levels for the rest of our bodies.[8] So if you do request your hormones to be checked, the TSH or even T4 tests are going to show you very little. And because you are most likely "in range," the doctor will usually make every effort to cover your symptoms with a prescription medication that treats your symptoms and not your root problem.

There are a lot of different hormone lab tests you can run, such as total testosterone, free testosterone, sex hormone binding globulin (SHBG), TSH, thyroid peroxidase (TPO) antibodies, free T3, reverse T3, free T4, progesterone level, and estradiol levels. Each tells you a bit more about your hormone levels, and these numbers are vital to understanding and treating your symptoms.

But a single test, especially the much-touted TSH test, is not going to tell you all that you need to know about your thyroid. You may need a full battery of hormone tests to find the real reasons behind your symptoms. The good news is that these tests exist. The bad news is that it may take some work to convince your doctor to get those tests done for you.

7. "A big study proved hormone treatment, especially estrogen, is bad for women and causes cancer and heart disease."

This is where, especially for women, the advances of hormone replacement therapy came to a grinding halt. The ramifications were global and deadly. The well-known US Women's Health Initiative was a study conducted by the National Institutes of Health (NIH) and included approximately 160,000 women. Part of what they wanted to know was if estrogen hormone treatment decreased or increased the risk of heart disease, cancer, and osteoporosis. The study began in 1991 and ran for fifteen years, but the hormone therapy components, which began in 1993, were stopped early because of the negative impact on those who participated. Indeed, there was an increased risk of heart attack, stroke, breast cancer, blood clots, and more.

THE NIH STUDY AND MASS HYSTERIA

The National Institutes of Health (NIH) began a ten-year prospective, double-blind placebo-controlled study in 1993 that was part of the Women's Health Initiative (WHI) to compare the effects of synthetic hormone replacement therapy using Premarin (estrogen) and Prempro (estrogen plus progestin) with dietary modifications and supplementation with calcium on cancer, heart disease, and osteoporosis. On

July 9, 2002, the estrogen-plus-progestin study was stopped early because the data showed an increased risk of heart attack, cancer, stroke, and blood clots in the women taking synthetic hormone replacement. Approximately 160,000 women were in the WHI study, and 16,000 were in the estrogen-plus-progestin part of the study. On average the women's age in the hormone arm of the study was sixty-three, or about ten years past menopause, which is much older than the average woman who starts hormone replacement. Many of the women also had preexisting conditions, including diabetes, osteoporosis, and heart disease, and many were smokers and did not follow a healthy diet or exercise.

The first part of the WHI study treated women with Prempro (a combination of Premarin and Provera). The results showed a significant increase in breast cancer, cardiovascular complications, and stroke. The second part of the WHI study treated women who had had hysterectomies with Premarin only. This part was also stopped early when women experienced an increased risk of stroke and did not show any cardiovascular benefits. The estrogen-only (Premarin) part of the study, however, showed a 23–33 percent decrease in breast cancer compared with controls.[9]

In 2002, as a direct result of the study, it was concluded that (1) Premarin and Provera increased the risk of heart disease, stroke, blood clots, breast cancer, and death when taken together; (2) Premarin increased the risk of heart disease, stroke, and blood clots but not breast cancer; and (3) there was no difference in the risk of heart disease. But doctors used this to scare millions of patients away from hormone replacement therapy. After all, why would you argue with facts?

MASS HYSTERIA CONTINUED

It's interesting—if estrogen or synthetic estrogen caused breast cancer, then why was the estrogen-only group in the NIH Women's Health Initiative showing a 23–33 percent decrease in breast cancer?

The media created significant hysteria throughout the nation with the unfounded fear that all hormones cause breast cancer, heart attacks, strokes, and blood clots when in reality the Provera, or synthetic progesterone, was the real culprit. Doctors and medical societies created even more panic fearing that they would be sued for prescribing the medications. As a result of the hormone scare, thousands of doctors quit prescribing hormone replacement and millions of women were thrown into hormone limbo and suffered from a lack of hormones. What they needed in truth was bioidentical hormone replacement taken in the form of transdermal cream, a patch, or a pellet instead of by mouth.

In fact, subsequent research has found that as many as 91,600 women died between 2002 and 2011 as a result of estrogen therapy avoidance![10]

Another study, which came out in 2013, estimates that somewhere between eighteen thousand and ninety-one thousand women died in the ten years that followed the abrupt almost complete cancellation of estrogen replacement therapy from diseases that could have been prevented by hormone replacement.[11]

When the doctors stopped prescribing estrogen, and the postmenopausal women quit taking estrogen to combat their menopausal symptoms (depression, weight gain, insomnia, irritability, and more), guess what happened? Those very symptoms returned with a vengeance!

It took another ten years before doctors, specialists, researchers, and patients began to question the findings. Not everything was adding up. It seemed that other undeniable facts and truths were running contrary to the study's findings.

Numerous new studies were initiated, and the old study was re-examined. What they found was not what the medical industry expected.

UNFORTUNATE FACT 1: *The estrogen hormone used in the study was Premarin.*

As we have discussed already, Premarin is a horse estrogen and one of the worst types of nonbioidentical hormones available. It is a combination of estrone and pregnant mare urine, with side effects that include heart attacks, blood clots, strokes, breast cancer, and more.

Why didn't those conducting the study use bioidentical hormones in the study, such as bioidentical estrogen and bioidentical progesterone instead of synthetic progesterone? To call all estrogen hormone therapy "cancer-causing" because they used one synthetic type is hardly a logical conclusion. Even worse, it is "scientifically wrong and dishonorable."[12] Obviously not all hormone drugs are created equal, so it was preposterous to call all hormones bad from one study using one synthetic hormone.

UNFORTUNATE FACT 2: *The women in the study were ten to twenty years past menopause. (The average age was sixty-three.)*

For best results, hormone therapy should be started shortly after menopause, but the ages of the women who participated were well past that. Many of the women already suffered from heart disease, blood clots, diabetes, osteoporosis, and other ailments, not to mention that many were overweight and smoked. Giving the wrong hormone to someone carrying a sickness would naturally lead to bad results, don't you think? They shut down the estrogen-plus-progestin study in 2002 and the estrogen-only study in 2004 for that very reason!

UNFORTUNATE FACT 3: *The estrogen (Premarin) was given orally, which is the least effective way to deliver estrogen into the body.*

Why didn't those conducting the study try to use some other delivery method instead of pills taken orally, such as shots, creams, pellets, or patches? Any estrogen taken by mouth can elevate the blood pressure, cause weight gain, and elevate triglycerides, which can increase the risk of heart disease.

Combine these three aspects together—(1) a nonbioidentical rather than a bioidentical hormone, (2) older women rather than a normal range of younger women in their fifties, and (3) an oral method rather than a pellet or transdermal—and the only result you could possibly get would be a bad one.

Surprise, surprise, the results were horrible. But because of this flawed study and subsequent faulty logic, it was quickly concluded that "estrogen causes breast cancer" and a laundry list of other terrible things.

There is no rewinding of the mass hysteria that followed the report's findings, but it is my hope—and the hope of many doctors, researchers, antiaging experts, and patients—that we will stick to the facts and leave faulty opinions at the door as we pursue health and wellness for us all.

8. "A big study proved hormone treatment is bad for men as well."

Men can certainly not be left out of the hormone confusion. In 2010 a study (called the TOM—Testosterone in Older Men with Mobility Limitations—study) was conducted in which men with low testosterone levels (below 350 ng/dL) were given testosterone therapy. Would the testosterone therapy increase their risks for stroke, heart attack, blood clots, testicular cancer, and death? That is certainly a valid question.

The TOM trial was done in frail elderly men with a high incidence of cardiovascular disease and other chronic diseases. It was stopped early due to increased cardiovascular events in the testosterone treatment group.

Then, in 2013, a retrospective cohort study of around eight thousand veterans with testosterone levels below 300 ng/dL was published in the *Journal of the American Medical Association* (*JAMA*). The study indicated that testosterone therapy was associated with an increased risk of adverse cardiovascular events.

IT'S A FACT

Muscle mass is the single greatest deterrent to the diseases of aging, and you need testosterone to get muscle mass.[13]

On the heels of the women's study, doctors were already scared. To make matters worse, lawyers jumped on the bandwagon and ran ads everywhere, encouraging men to sue their doctors if they had been given testosterone therapy. Naturally hormone therapy for men took a dive.

However, it wasn't long before both the TOM study and the *JAMA* study were criticized. The TOM study was a randomized, placebo-controlled, double-blind trial, but it only had 209 participants, and many of the participants were already at high risk for cardiovascular events—of the participants who used the testosterone gel, 85 percent had high blood pressure, 53 percent had preexisting cardiovascular disease, 45 percent were obese, 24 percent had diabetes, and 74 percent were current or former smokers. In addition, estradiol levels were not monitored, and excess estrogen increases the risk of blood clots.[14] Also, the study used a gel testosterone only. But the most significant factor was that everyone was over sixty-five years of age.

When you have men over sixty-five who have testosterone levels lower than 350 ng/dL, you are talking to a bunch of men who already have or are at very high risk for heart attacks, diabetes, prediabetes, osteoporosis, sarcopenia, obesity, autoimmune diseases, blood clots, strokes, prostate cancer, dementia, Alzheimer's, Parkinson's, and much more.

Then there was the *JAMA* study. It was a cohort study, not a randomized, placebo-controlled, double-blind trial. Of the 8,709 veterans included in the study, approximately 20 percent had already had a heart attack, 50 percent had diabetes, and over 80 percent already had coronary artery disease. In addition, estradiol levels were not reported. However, the most significant factor calling into question the results of the study is that the testosterone level of the patients who received testosterone therapy averaged 332 ng/dL.[15]

The optimal range of testosterone to offer cardioprotection or protection against a heart attack is a testosterone level of 500–900 ng/dL. The testosterone level reached by the patients in the *JAMA* study was well below this range.

The TOM study and the *JAMA* study vilified testosterone and falsely claimed it increased heart attack risks in men. These studies have caused confusion and fear similar to the Women's Health Initiative in 2002. But experts found that both of these studies are severely flawed and limited.[16] Testosterone is protective to the heart, and considerable data and studies show it does not increase the risk of heart attack or stroke. Low testosterone and suboptimal testosterone are actually what have been associated with increased incidence of heart disease and death.[17] And interestingly a retrospective cohort study in 2015, this time of over eighty-three thousand veterans with low testosterone levels, found that normalization of testosterone levels is associated with a reduction in heart attacks and other cardiovascular events.[18]

Giving a glass of water to a dying man does not prove the water was bad! Nor does giving testosterone therapy to sick men prove that testosterone causes their ailments, even death. Testosterone has been proved time and again to be both useful and necessary for men and women.

One of the top urologists in the world, Abraham Morgentaler, was one of many who questioned the study and went about doing research of his own. He found that men with low testosterone often have undiagnosed prostate cancer. The cancer rates are the same between those with low or normal levels of testosterone, but the symptoms of low testosterone seem to mask the cancer. Then when they do get checked, the prostate cancer is usually more advanced. Low testosterone is to blame, not normal or optimal levels of testosterone.[19] Prostate cancer occurs more commonly when testosterone levels are low.

CONTROVERSIES COMING INTO THE LIGHT

There have been controversies around all the hormones, especially estrogen, progesterone, and testosterone. Do they cause cancers, heart attacks, blood clots, and a host of other ailments?

No, the bioidentical hormones do not.[20] But to clarify the statement even more, I tell patients hormone replacement therapy does not cause cancers, disease, or sickness, or even increase your risks for them—when you optimize your hormones using bioidentical hormones with the right delivery system. The truth is, these same bioidentical hormones, specifically estrogen, progesterone, and testosterone, have been shown time and time again to actually prevent cancer, heart disease, heart attacks, and much more. And when your hormone levels are optimized, your body is usually the healthiest it can be. A low testosterone level, even if it's in the low normal range, still increases your risk for heart disease.[21]

I wouldn't be surprised if testosterone is going to be part of the answer to Alzheimer's. Why? The use of testosterone in older men has already been found to slow and sometimes stop the progression of Alzheimer's![22] In fact, maintaining healthy testosterone levels may even prevent Alzheimer's disease.[23] Similarly estrogen has been shown to prevent heart disease, osteoporosis, strokes, and memory-related diseases, including dementia and Alzheimer's.

Put the fears to rest. Close the door on confusion. Bioidentical hormones are not going to shorten your life. If anything, they will help you live longer, help you enjoy your life as you have always envisioned, and help keep you disease resistant.

CHAPTER 3

SYMPTOMS OF HORMONES OUT OF BALANCE

F OR MY WIFE, Mary, the Keto Zone diet (as described in my previous book, *Dr. Colbert's Keto Zone Diet*) worked great. The low-carb, high–healthy fat, medium-protein diet burned off excess fat, decreased her aches and pains, and boosted her energy levels. Add in a simple exercise program, and she lost ten to fifteen pounds within a few short months and kept the weight off.

But the biggest boost for her was the hormone replacement therapy. When we optimized her hormone levels (especially her testosterone and thyroid), gone were the cold hands and cold feet, the occasional brain fog, and afternoon tiredness. Instead, her metabolism went into high gear, tiredness disappeared, and an additional ten pounds melted right off.

She couldn't believe it, but when we brought her hormone levels up to what they are with a twenty-year-old woman, the change was almost instant. "I haven't felt so good or had so much energy in years," she told me.

I've done the same thing myself, optimized my hormone levels to what they were when I was around twenty years old. I always try to take care of my body, eat according to the Keto Zone diet, go to the gym a lot, and live a healthy lifestyle, but optimizing my hormones was an incredible change. You could say, metaphorically speaking, it was like someone turned on the lights. I could see before, but I didn't know how dark it was in the room until the lights went on.

For me, it was my thyroid. It was not low, but it was definitely suboptimal. This is often described as a "sluggish" thyroid. It still works, more puttering than purring, but symptoms develop that do not go away on their own. The cold hands and cold feet were a telltale sign, along with afternoon tiredness. When I optimized my thyroid with natural thyroid hormones, the bothersome symptoms disappeared completely.

For me, there was something more. My dad died of Alzheimer's disease, and the fact that testosterone replacement therapy helps prevent, stop, and delay Alzheimer's is good enough reason to keep my hormone levels optimized for the rest of my life.

Today, Mary and I both have more energy than we know what to do with. There is no room for depression or lethargy when you are high on living, and we like it that way. We only wish we had started earlier!

It would take a very long time to list all the benefits that come from hormone replacement therapy and optimizing people's hormone levels. I know how it has benefited me, Mary, my brother, my mom, and many patients over the years.

How it will benefit you depends on your body and your needs, but I can promise you that when your light switch turns on, you will never be the same! Feel free to write me and tell me about it. (Maybe I'll be able to use your story in other books or blog posts.) The beautiful thing will be the fact that you can actually enjoy these symptoms. When the bad symptoms of low hormone levels are replaced by good symptoms, it's a beautiful day!

WHAT ARE YOUR SYMPTOMS?

Symptoms, whether they are good or bad, are a reflection or echo of what is already happening inside our bodies. Everything we eat, drink, breathe, touch, experience, believe, and choose to do *today* will be reflected in our bodies *tomorrow* and in the days to come. That means the symptoms you have today are the result of the many yesterdays that lead up to this point. It also means that doing something different today will bring about a different tomorrow as well!

Is this not exactly the principle from Scripture of sowing and reaping?

> For whatever a man sows, that he will also reap.
> —GALATIANS 6:7

This always holds true. It is a fact of life. Thankfully when we sow good seeds, we also reap good rewards in return.

IT'S A FACT

A suboptimal, sluggish, but still "in range" thyroid usually means constipation, obesity, fatigue, cold hands, cold feet, slow metabolism, hair loss, and more, and many doctors misdiagnose it.

So what are your symptoms? Every doctor visit begins there. But what do the symptoms mean? And is there something you can really do about your persistent symptoms? If you have suffered from reoccurring symptoms, you are desperate for answers. I have met people who have put on a brave face and soldiered through ten, twenty, thirty, even forty years of some pretty discouraging symptoms. Years! Without real answers, the symptoms will persist. But do you really want to wait that long before you get help?

Below is an alphabetized list of hormone-related symptoms and diseases that I see every single day. Every doctor does. These may also be the very symptoms you are dealing with right now. Maybe you are looking for help, trying to find answers, and getting increasingly frustrated at how hard it is to break free.

Take a few minutes to look through this list. As you do, rate the degree that the symptoms affect you. The list and the rating system will help bring clarity to your own unique situation. Later in the book we will explore these hormone-related issues and what you can do about them.

SYMPTOM	RATE IT			
	0 (NEVER)	1 (OCCASIONALLY)	2 (OFTEN)	3 (ALWAYS)
Absence of morning erection	0	1	2	3
Absence of zest for life	0	1	2	3
Achy joints	0	1	2	3
Acne as an adult	0	1	2	3
Alzheimer's	0	1	2	3
Arthritis	0	1	2	3
Autoimmune disorder	0	1	2	3
Belly fat	0	1	2	3

SYMPTOM	RATE IT			
	0 (NEVER)	1 (OCCASIONALLY)	2 (OFTEN)	3 (ALWAYS)
Bladder infection/leak	0	1	2	3
Bone loss	0	1	2	3
Brain fog	0	1	2	3
Brittle nails	0	1	2	3
Carpal tunnel syndrome	0	1	2	3
Cellulite	0	1	2	3
Chronic infections	0	1	2	3
Cold backside	0	1	2	3
Cold hands/feet	0	1	2	3
Cold intolerance	0	1	2	3
Concentration difficulty	0	1	2	3
Constipation	0	1	2	3
Dementia	0	1	2	3
Depression	0	1	2	3
Diabetes (type 2)	0	1	2	3
Dizziness	0	1	2	3
Dry eyes	0	1	2	3
Dry skin	0	1	2	3
Enlarged prostate	0	1	2	3
Erectile dysfunction	0	1	2	3
Excessive earwax	0	1	2	3
Exhaustion	0	1	2	3
Facial hair increase	0	1	2	3
Fatigue	0	1	2	3
Fatty clavicles	0	1	2	3
Fibromyalgia	0	1	2	3
Fluid retention	0	1	2	3
Food cravings	0	1	2	3
Forgetfulness	0	1	2	3
Frailty	0	1	2	3
Frequent illness	0	1	2	3
Frequent naps	0	1	2	3
Frequent UTIs	0	1	2	3

SYMPTOM	RATE IT			
	0 (NEVER)	1 (OCCASIONALLY)	2 (OFTEN)	3 (ALWAYS)
Goiter	0	1	2	3
Grumpiness	0	1	2	3
Hair breakage	0	1	2	3
Hair loss	0	1	2	3
Hard/round stools	0	1	2	3
Heart disease	0	1	2	3
Heart palpitations	0	1	2	3
Heavy periods	0	1	2	3
High blood pressure	0	1	2	3
High cholesterol	0	1	2	3
High cortisol levels	0	1	2	3
High insulin levels	0	1	2	3
Hoarse, husky voice	0	1	2	3
Hypoglycemia	0	1	2	3
IBS	0	1	2	3
Infertility	0	1	2	3
Infrequent sexual climax	0	1	2	3
Insomnia	0	1	2	3
Irritability	0	1	2	3
Lack of sex drive	0	1	2	3
Light-headedness	0	1	2	3
Loss of curves	0	1	2	3
Loss of energy	0	1	2	3
Loss of enjoyment	0	1	2	3
Loss of stamina	0	1	2	3
Low body temperature	0	1	2	3
Lupus	0	1	2	3
Man boobs	0	1	2	3
Migraines	0	1	2	3
Miscarriages	0	1	2	3
Mood swings	0	1	2	3
Muscle loss	0	1	2	3
Muscle pain	0	1	2	3

SYMPTOM	RATE IT			
	0 (NEVER)	1 (OCCASIONALLY)	2 (OFTEN)	3 (ALWAYS)
Muscle weakness	0	1	2	3
Nausea	0	1	2	3
Nervousness	0	1	2	3
Obesity	0	1	2	3
Osteoporosis	0	1	2	3
Panic attacks	0	1	2	3
Parkinson's	0	1	2	3
Poor memory	0	1	2	3
Prediabetes	0	1	2	3
Puffy/bags under eyes	0	1	2	3
Ridged nails	0	1	2	3
Ringing in the ears	0	1	2	3
Sagging breasts	0	1	2	3
Salt craving	0	1	2	3
Sarcopenia	0	1	2	3
Scleroderma	0	1	2	3
Skin wrinkles	0	1	2	3
Slow metabolism	0	1	2	3
Strokes	0	1	2	3
Sweating	0	1	2	3
Sweet craving	0	1	2	3
Swollen jawline	0	1	2	3
Thinning eyebrows	0	1	2	3
Thinning skin	0	1	2	3
Tremors	0	1	2	3
Turned down lip corners	0	1	2	3
Vaginal dryness	0	1	2	3
Weight gain	0	1	2	3
Worse allergies	0	1	2	3

Many of these symptoms or diseases are progressive in that if you don't treat them successfully, they continue to worsen over time. That only makes sense, unfortunately. To make matters worse, these symptoms and diseases are also usually interconnected, which means one thing leads to the next and the next and the next. This also usually gets worse as you age.

Take obesity, for example. Statistics show that about 40 percent of Americans are now classified as obese.[1] I have been watching this trend for decades, and the percentage is only going up.

Of course obesity is not entirely a hormone-related issue, but low testosterone levels certainly do speed up obesity. But that is not all. The low testosterone levels are also causing depression, high cholesterol, heart disease, a lack of sex drive, muscle loss, bone loss, diabetes, and much more in both men and women. And this will only get worse because obesity drives testosterone levels lower, which only adds more weight, and it all spirals ever downward.

Do you want to know how many major diseases follow obesity? It is thirty-five and counting! You read that correctly. The ever-rising obesity rates are triggering the onslaught of thirty-five other epidemics.

Stop for a second and consider the cost of all that. It was estimated a few years back that by 2030 the cost of these preventable diseases will be close to fifty trillion dollars![2] Sadly you read that right, but it is all preventable!

SOLUTIONS TO YOUR SYMPTOMS

Most doctors will look at your symptoms and, based on what they were taught in medical school and by the pharmaceutical reps, give you a prescription to manage your symptoms. The root cause is seldom addressed. The proof is in your body: Did the symptom go away or not? That fact is pretty easy to measure.

As symptoms persist, patients return again and again to their doctors for help, but if nothing changes, their frustration grows. Patients hope desperately that someone will come up with an answer before their symptoms drive them crazy! I understand the frustration of having symptoms and not finding the cure. It took me many years to find the root cause of my psoriasis. I was an itchy, scratching, painful mess in the meantime.

The ratio of women to men in all cases of thyroid disease: 3 to 1.[3]

Looking back at the long list of symptoms, how many of them describe how you feel or match your own concerns? Granted, the list runs from A to Z and includes some very scary diseases, but let me tell you something else: every symptom on this list has a direct link to your body's hormone levels. In most cases, bioidentical hormone replacement therapy can get to the root cause of the symptoms.

That is incredible news! I see it happen every day. It's exciting, it's real, and it's helping people deal with their symptoms so they can move on with life. For example, I have had hundreds of young women who had low free T3 (a thyroid hormone) levels come to my offices over the years with the complaint that they couldn't get pregnant. When we optimized their thyroid and brought up their T3 levels, they got pregnant!

Their frustration turned into incredible gladness. I have often thought this was an exact parallel to "Weeping may endure for a night, but joy comes in the morning" (Ps. 30:5).

It happens all the time. When people optimize their hormone levels, symptoms usually disappear and sickness usually goes away.

I have found that balancing hormones will also usually take away most symptoms, which is amazing. But to slow the aging process, to stop disease in its tracks, to rebuild muscle and bone, to burn off that stubborn belly fat, to wipe away wrinkles, and so much more, you must optimize—not just balance—your hormone levels. The process is easy.

"How effective is it?" patients ask me. Others have little hope of getting free of their symptoms when they tell me, "I've dealt with this for over twenty years."

If you came into my office with any of these symptoms and we got your hormones optimized, I would be very surprised if your symptoms were not completely erased in six to twelve months. I mean that! And a full year later you may not even recognize yourself in the mirror. I have had patients come in for a checkup and laugh, telling me how much fun it is to hear people say, "What have you been doing to yourself?" or "What are you eating?" or "Please tell me your secret!"

I had one patient who literally turned back time. She looked at least twenty years older than she really was due to her wrinkly skin (a symptom of hormone imbalance). But when we optimized her hormones, her skin regained its youthful appearance and many of her wrinkles disappeared. Suddenly she looked twenty years younger! Her friends were awestruck, wondering what she had done.

Though the list of symptoms was long and daunting, know that whatever your symptom, with optimized hormones it just might be a thing of the past!

CHAPTER 4

WHAT IS HAPPENING TO OUR HORMONES?

NOT LONG AGO a new patient named Betty came to my office. Betty had been battling hormone issues for quite some time. Based on her blood work showing high thyroid antibodies (TPO) and low free T3, it looked as if she had Hashimoto's thyroiditis, the most common cause of low thyroid in the country.

"My endocrinologist looked at those numbers too," she explained. "He said we should not treat it until it gets really bad."

That was unfortunate advice because hormonal problems, especially Hashimoto's, are like a fuse. Once lit, it is very hard to put out. That is because Hashimoto's is an autoimmune disorder, and her own immune system was forming antibodies to attack her thyroid. The longer that continued, the greater the damage, and eventually her body would destroy her thyroid.

Hashimoto's thyroiditis, discovered in 1912 by a Japanese doctor named Hakuro Hashimoto, is an autoimmune disease. It is sometimes difficult to diagnose because as the thyroid is dying, it sometimes spurts out extra thyroid and sometimes little to none at all. Basically it flips and flops, sometimes giving you symptoms of being hyperthyroid (where your thyroid is producing too much thyroid hormone) and sometimes hypothyroid (where your thyroid is not producing enough thyroid hormone).

"But when your thyroid is eventually destroyed, you are definitely going to be hypothyroid," I explained.

"So what do I do?" Betty asked. "How do we know for sure that it's Hashimoto's?"

The answer was by measuring the antibodies that were attacking her thyroid. That is the most concrete way to confirm the symptoms. The two antibodies that you can test for are thyroid peroxidase

35

(TPOAbs) and thyroglobulin (TgAbs). Interestingly your body can have these antibodies doing damage to your thyroid long before you develop symptoms of Hashimoto's. That is another strong reason why optimizing hormones is a smart move.

What quantity of antibodies are we really talking about anyway? According to Izabella Wentz, in her book *Hashimoto's Thyroiditis: Lifestyle Interventions for Finding and Treating the Root Cause*, the following amounts of TPO antibodies tell the degree of Hashimoto's that someone might have:

Above 30 IU/mL: The person may have Hashimoto's.

Under 100 IU/mL: Hashimoto's is not yet at hypothyroidism levels.

Over 500 IU/mL: The person's Hashimoto's is aggressive.[1]

The antibody tests showed the amount of antibodies in Betty's system. Her numbers were just under 100 IU/mL. She was sliding into Hashimoto's all right, but her thyroid was still puttering along.

IT'S A FACT

Iodine deficiency can cause hypothyroidism and goiters and is the leading cause of hypothyroidism in many under-developed countries. However, Hashimoto's—not iodine deficiency—is the leading cause of hypothyroidism in the United States and European countries that supplement iodine intake by adding it to salt and foods. In fact, Hashimoto's is responsible for 90 percent of hypothyroidism cases in the United States.[2]

When it comes to Hashimoto's, there is much debate about iodine and the TPO antibodies. Iodine deficiency can contribute to Hashimoto's, and iodine excess can also contribute to Hashimoto's thyroiditis. Although rare, it is selenium that we in North America are usually deficient in, as well as iodine.

Iodine is important for thyroid health, but I first treat Hashimoto's patients with selenium (selenomethionine, 200 mcg a day) for four to six weeks to give their thyroid the protection it needs. The powerful antioxidant glutathione peroxidase requires selenium to protect the thyroid cells from hydrogen peroxide produced by the inflamed thyroid.

That is where we began with Betty. First was selenium, a supplement available at most health food stores, and then we moved to optimize her thyroid hormone levels. Within a few short months, she noticed an improvement with her symptoms. And when we ran her blood work the next time, her TPO antibodies had already decreased significantly. I also placed her on a gluten-free diet. Gluten is a common trigger for Hashimoto's thyroiditis.

Betty's thyroid may never fully recover (though I have seen it commonly happen), but by optimizing her thyroid hormone levels and giving her selenium and a gluten-free diet, she is well on her way to living life without any Hashimoto's symptoms.

THE TOP SIX HORMONE DISRUPTORS

Several years ago I wrote the book *Toxic Relief,* and even then I was amazed at the thousands of toxic chemicals that we are exposed to on a regular basis in the air, water, and food. Approximately seventy thousand chemicals are in use in the United States, only a tiny fraction of which have been fully tested for their ability to cause harm to health and the environment.[3] Now, in the twenty-first century, everyone (even a newborn baby) carries a toxic burden. The Environmental Working Group examined the umbilical cord blood of ten newborns of various ethnicities, such as African American, Asian, and Hispanic. The blood samples from the newborns had as many as 232 chemicals.[4]

IT'S A FACT

Iodine is in many foods, including yogurt, cow's milk, eggs, strawberries, mozzarella cheese, sea veggies (kelp, dulse, nori), multivitamins with iodine, iodized salt, saltwater fish, shellfish, and more.

I call certain toxic chemicals "hormone disruptors" because they disturb your endocrine system, confusing your hormonal systems—including the thyroid, adrenal, pituitary, and sex hormones—which then may cause either an increase or decrease in the production of different hormones. This wreaks havoc on your hormones and creates hormone imbalances that contribute to breast cancer, reproductive problems, infertility, decreased sperm count, ADD, ADHD, autism, slow cognitive development, changes in metabolism, weight gain, lower sex hormones, immune disorders, decreased thyroid function, and lower IQs.

In this world you are surrounded by endocrine disruptors that try to work their way in and create havoc in your body. Some disruptors you would expect; others are not so obvious, but all of them slowly chip away at your overall health. The basic principle is this: fewer disruptors means a healthier body. Virtually all disruptors are interconnected. This means decreasing the number of disruptions will increase your health, and when you remove one disruptor, it brings with it an avalanche of other good side effects. Here are the top hormone disruptors, in random order, along with ways you can minimize the disruption or stop it from taking place in your body.

Disruptor 1—lifestyle and choices

The lifestyle you choose to live certainly counts as one of those "I expected to hear that" types of hormone disruptors. Whether it is weight gain, a lack of exercise, extra stress, anger and unforgiveness, drinking too much alcohol, or some other thing that can be controlled, each of these negatively affects your hormone levels.

And as your hormone levels drop, you get symptoms (such as those on the long list in the previous chapter) that mirror the problem. That is the beginning of the slow slide toward even more symptoms and poorer health. I have seen a lot of people leave an office job for a more physically demanding job and suddenly lose twenty to fifty pounds. They had not realized it at the time, but their previous lifestyle and choices were setting them up for hormone disruption.

The answer is what you would expect: make better choices, maintain your exercise program, eat healthier, relax more, and so on, but it is completely true. The whole obesity epidemic, for example, and the thirty-five major diseases that follow it, is mostly based on the choices we make.

Men of today have about 20 percent less testosterone than men did just twenty years ago.[5]

When your lifestyle and choices are healthy, they are also hormone-friendly, and that dramatically decreases the chances of having any hormone deficiency symptoms.

Disruptor 2—medications

A few years ago a study by Johns Hopkins University found that medical errors were the United States' third-leading cause of death.[6] Medical mistakes cause a lot of deaths—250,000 a year, according to the JHU study—but how many other medical errors, in the form of wrong diagnoses and side effects from medications, lead to a life of incredible pain, misery, discomfort, fatigue, and unnecessary expenses? And when you consider the fact that the medications affect the body's cells, it only makes sense that one of the greatest hormone disruptors is the medication we take as prescribed!

A few years ago the second-most-prescribed drug in America was a cholesterol-lowering statin drug.[7] Some of the side effects of statin medication include liver damage, muscle pain and damage, neurological side effects such as confusion and memory loss, and elevated blood sugar or type 2 diabetes.[8] Statin drugs also lower testosterone levels. Add to that the fact that a huge portion of Americans are taking anti-depressant medications, which also usually decrease testosterone levels.

Combined, I estimate that 55 percent of the entire US population is taking pills that directly and negatively affect hormone levels. The nation's ever-increasing rates of obesity and many diseases simply reflect our increasing medication rates.

Generally speaking, the more medicated a nation is, the greater the level of hormone disruption. As I mentioned in an earlier chapter, almost 70 percent of Americans are taking at least one prescription medication, according to a 2013 Mayo Clinic study.

Disruptor 3—things you touch

No, I am not talking about people who work in a chemical factory. This applies to everyone, and you may be surprised to discover just how many things you touch that negatively affect your hormone levels. That is because the chemicals get into your body through your skin, accumulate, and eventually may cause long-term damage. Here is a short list of some of the disruptors you touch and how they affect you:

Ever heard of BPA plastic (bisphenol A)? It was discovered in 1891 and was one of those "breakthrough" creations that were great at the time but came back to really bite us in the end. Since the 1950s BPA has been used to harden plastic and make epoxy resin. Among other uses, BPA can be found in the lining of food and beverage containers. It is still in production. Currently more than a million pounds of BPA are released into the environment each year.[9]

What does BPA do to your body? It is an environmental estrogen and behaves like estrogen in the body. BPA is in most canned foods as BPA-based lining, but it is also in aluminum beverage cans, aerosol cans for whipped toppings and nonstick spray, and the lids of many glass jar items, plastic bottles, and dental materials (such as dental sealants).

Specifically BPA has been found to cause or contribute to cancer, fertility problems, miscarriages, diabetes, development issues, early onset of puberty in girls, heart disease, and a decreased sperm count in men. It also plays an expected role with the obesity epidemic because it wreaks havoc on our metabolism and our insulin levels.[10] Over time it increases our body mass index and belly fat[11] and makes our fat cells fatter, which naturally increases obesity.[12] If that isn't enough, BPA increases the risk of other health disorders, such as type 2 diabetes, heart disease, and behavioral problems.[13]

Believe it or not, most of the BPA we come in contact with is in our pantries and refrigerators. It is found in the coating on the inside of metal-canned foods and in the plastic containers we store or heat our food in. It was in baby formula bottles, but that was banned. (If you are wondering why it would be banned from baby products but allowed to continue to be used on the rest of us, I'm wondering that as well.) BPA is estimated to be in 75 percent of canned foods in North America, and while some cans are "BPA-free," if they have been coated with a similar chemical (BPS), it is best to avoid them as well.[14]

What should you do? I recommend all the time to patients to buy glass jars of food rather than canned food and store food at home in ceramic containers. Cooking or reheating in those containers is then safe without worry of increasing BPA exposure.

There is another source of BPA that affects us all: cash register receipts. Most receipts contain BPA.[15] If your hands are moist, that increases the BPA transfer. And as you would expect, paper money has BPA because it touches receipts in wallets.[16] Researchers recently reported that male factory workers in China who were exposed to significant BPA levels experienced sexual problems, including erectile dysfunction.[17]

Ever heard of phthalates? You have, but by another name. It is often listed simply as "fragrance" in the ingredients of your soaps, perfumes, laundry detergents, cosmetics, and moisturizers. There are about ten different types of phthalates in commercial use as plasticizers, solvents, antifoam agents, and alcohol denaturants.[18]

Phthalates used as plasticizers make plastics more flexible, but the adverse effect is that they cause males to become more feminized.[19] Phthalates are found in soft plastic flooring, food packaging, shower curtains, household cleaners, cosmetics and personal care products, and even some toys. They even are outgassed from flooring, furniture, mattresses, and upholstery.

To reduce your exposure to phthalates:

- Install glass shower doors, and get rid of shower curtains.
- Use natural brands of toothpaste, shampoos, and cosmetics.
- Get rid of scented candles, air fresheners, dryer sheets, and synthetic fragrances.
- Use glass instead of plastic to store food.
- Use natural cleaning products.
- Do not let your children drink from a garden hose, which is made from phthalate plastics.
- Filter the tap water in your home.

As a disruptor, phthalates negatively affect our (both men's and women's) ability to use the testosterone that is in our bodies. All of us, men and women, need testosterone, and if we cannot use it correctly, the effects are usually going to be seen in decreased muscle mass, decreased libido, and an increased risk of depression, weight gain, man boobs, erectile dysfunction, and memory problems.

Heard of parabens? These are in shampoos, lotions, and body washes. They are often used as preservatives that prevent mold and yeast from growing in pharmaceuticals, toiletries, and cosmetics.[20] Parabens can cause skin irritation and interfere with hormones, especially estrogen.

How about triclosan? It has been banned in soap in the United States but is found in some shaving gel, deodorants, and even certain toothpastes. This disruptor interferes with your thyroid hormones.

Disruptor 4—things you eat

You might find it hard to believe that things you touch can cause negative effects on your hormones. What you put in your mouth is another matter entirely. Remember the BPA that is in canned foods, plastic containers, and receipts? It is also in water. Not long ago a groundwater test across the United States found approximately 30 percent of test samples contained BPA.[21]

In addition, many pesticides, herbicides, and insecticides that farmers use to grow food end up going straight into our bodies, and they can directly affect our thyroids.[22] But it doesn't need to be a bug spray to hurt your hormones. Did you know that infants given soy baby formula are nearly three times as likely to develop antithyroid antibodies as breastfed babies?[23]

Heard of DDT (dichlorodiphenyltrichloroethane)? As a nation we used DDT heavily for about thirty years as an insecticide. It is great at killing mosquitos, but it messes with several different hormones, including thyroid, testosterone, and estrogen. DDT was banned in the US in 1972, but many third-world countries still use it to fight mosquitoes and malaria, and it ends up in the countries' food supply that may be exported to our country. DDT is still in the soil, air, and food and water supply, and it eventually ends up in our bodies.

Heard of PFOA (perfluorooctanoic acid)? This synthetic chemical is known for its grease- and stain-repelling properties as well as its heat resistance, which is why it's used to make cookware nonstick, furniture flame-retardant, carpets stain-resistant, and clothing waterproof.[24] PFOA can affect thyroid and sex hormone levels. Our bodies store these toxins, and over time, even decades, these toxins prove toxic to our bodies. It is usually your hormones and thyroid that pay a price for it all.

Disruptor 5—deficiencies

The standard American diet is usually low in certain key nutrients that support a healthy thyroid. Optimal conversion of the inactive T4 thyroid hormone to the active T3 thyroid hormone requires a ferritin level of about 90–100 ng/mL. We measure iron stores by checking the ferritin level, and if the ferritin level is low, the thyroid function is usually sluggish or compromised. Low iron is a primary reason why premenopausal women lose their hair. A ferritin level of 40 ng/mL usually stops hair loss, and a level of 70 ng/mL starts regrowing hair.[25]

About 90 percent of the patients I've checked are low in iodine. I switch them from table salt to sea salt or Himalayan salt, which contain iodine, and usually start an iodine supplement unless they have Hashimoto's thyroiditis. If they have Hashimoto's, I always start with selenium first and add iodine after two months; otherwise the iodine could worsen the Hashimoto's. If the patient has Hashimoto's, you can bet he or she is usually low in selenium. I place the patient on selenomethionine at 200 mcg per day. Also, optimizing vitamin D_3 levels to 50–80 ng/mL helps prevent all autoimmune diseases, including Hashimoto's thyroiditis.

Bromine in most white bread served in restaurants will compete with iodine and may compromise optimal thyroid function. Chlorine and fluoride will also compete with iodine, as will mercury from dental amalgam, in many types of fish, and from breathing air from coal-burning power plants.

Unexpectedly some vegetables in their raw state can block iodine uptake into the thyroid, which then may reflect the symptoms you would have with hypothyroidism. This includes veggies such as raw broccoli, cauliflower, bok choy, cabbage, and others.[26] The answer is to cook or steam the vegetables. If you do eat them raw, stick to small amounts of these veggies.

Disruptor 6—aging

For women, around age forty their levels of testosterone usually begin to decline. Then five to ten years later, their progesterone usually starts to slide, followed five years later by their estrogen beginning to decline.

For men, their testosterone levels begin to drop after age thirty, and by the time they are around forty-five to fifty, many have become "grumpy old men" because of low testosterone. When testosterone reaches low enough levels, other hormones, such as DHEA and adrenal hormones, are usually also low. Estradiol may stay low or rise in low testosterone men.

At age fifty our hormone levels usually go down dramatically, and when our hormones drop, the liver usually revs up cholesterol production in an effort to make more sex hormones from cholesterol, and that is one of the reasons why cholesterol levels begin to go up around age fifty. Cholesterol-lowering drugs are usually prescribed at this point, but they lower testosterone all the more.

IT'S A FACT

When you optimize your hormones, your cholesterol level usually drops. The bad (LDL) cholesterol numbers usually go down, and the good (HDL) cholesterol numbers usually go up. For people over fifty this is especially important.

The process of aging is gradual, but it does not stop for any of us. Yes, it can be accelerated by the many endocrine disruptors we have already mentioned (also, stress, a chronic illness, or menopause/a hysterectomy can speed up aging), but it is a gradual process that cannot be stopped completely by diet, pills, or exercise.

We are told to accept the sagging features, expanding waistlines, and reduced muscle tone because "that's what happens when you get older." Even irritability, a lack of libido, and depression are included in the "getting old" package.

The effects of aging, like the other disruptors, can be slowed or stopped and sometimes reversed when we optimize our hormones.

Mix It All Together

All these different hormone disruptors can be chipping away at our hormone levels at the same time. Apart from the symptoms, which are too often misdiagnosed, usually we are completely unaware of what is happening.

A good example of this combination of disruptors at work is seen with gynecomastia (the enlarging of men's breasts, or "man boobs"). The increased incidence of this, of course, follows the decrease of testosterone and addition of belly and chest fat, but there is a list of medications, drugs, and products that also cause it.[27] These include:

- antianxiety meds
- heart meds
- ulcer meds
- antibiotics
- tricyclic antidepressants
- glucocorticoid steroids
- anabolic steroids
- antiandrogens (for treating prostate cancer)
- cancer treatment
- alcohol
- marijuana
- heroin
- amphetamines

Hormone disruptors do plenty of damage when they are alone, but when they team up, they cause even more havoc. The combined effect may be why men's average sperm count has dropped 50 percent in less than forty years.[28]

Not only are the effects of all these disruptors (medications, chemicals, aging, poor life choices, and so on) depressing to think about, they actually cause depression, along with countless other ailments, such as type 2 diabetes, high blood pressure, prediabetes, heart disease, obesity, insulin resistance, insomnia, and so much more.

But there is good news! I have seen every single one of these symptoms reversed with many patients who optimized their hormones. I have seen people eventually get off the medications they hate and that cause numerous side effects. When you optimize your hormone levels, you enable all your systems to function optimally. And what is more, optimizing your hormones is the absolute best way to fight aging.

We all can rejoice with that!

PART II
MAKING HORMONES WORK FOR YOU

P ART 2 BEGINS with the foundation of all hormone health, then outlines a practical example of how hormone therapy can work for you, regardless of your symptoms, diseases, or concerns. The final chapter works through many of the questions that new patients have as they consider bioidentical hormone therapy.

CHAPTER 5

THE FOUNDATION OF YOUR HORMONE HEALTH

T ERRANCE HAD LOW testosterone and low thyroid. At least that was his guess. His once athletic body was getting increasingly fat around the middle, he had needed to buy new pants twice as his waistline expanded, his stamina and drive were noticeably decreased, and he noticed some inabilities at home with his wife that he didn't really want to discuss with anyone.

The worst for him was how he felt. He described his body, energy levels, and gumption with words like *sluggish, slow,* and *feeling down, grumpy, and irritable.* He had prided himself in his after-hours work on other money-making hobbies, such as reupholstering furniture for his growing list of clients, but it had been many months since he had enough energy to do anything extra.

"It's just the stress I'm under," he had told himself. That was about a year ago, and his new job, with a lengthy commute, was not showing any signs of calming down. His wife encouraged him to get his hormone levels checked, and he did. It was his testosterone and thyroid levels that he wanted to see the most. The results confirmed his hunch:

Total T: 351 ng/dL (nanograms per deciliter)

Free T3: 2.5 pg/mL (picograms per milliliter)

His numbers, accounting for the natural loss of testosterone and thyroid in men over time, matched those of a seventy- or eighty-year-old man. Needless to say, at age thirty-five Terrance was not too pleased.

According to the Endocrine Society, the range for total T in non-obese men ages nineteen through thirty-nine is 264–916 ng/dL.[1] (It was 348–1197 ng/dL for many years before it was recently lowered.) I recommend men have their total T at 500 ng/dL or higher, but when we optimize their hormone levels, we aim for 900–1100 ng/dL (the typical range of a twenty-five-year-old). The range for free T3, according to LabCorp, is 2.0–4.4 pg/mL.[2] At 2.5 pg/mL, Terrance was at the low end of normal.

"I don't want to feel like I'm eighty! I'm only thirty-five!" he complained.

He felt he was too young to begin hormone therapy, though his body certainly needed it. Based on averages, his weight and symptoms put him right in the middle of normal for most people in the United States. He was the normal average, and yet he did not feel good, nor was he very proud of how he looked.

We discussed it, and he decided he wanted to get his body back in shape, eat better foods, and try to bring up his hormone levels on his own. He was motivated to make a change because he knew where he was going if he didn't change course now.

So he began.

THE FOUNDATIONAL DIY PLAN

The foundational do-it-yourself plan is really the best place for most people, regardless of age or gender, to begin their hormone replacement therapy journey. It is the basis of good health, and without the good and necessary habits it brings, optimizing hormones without the foundation in place takes more time, effort, and money.

Terrance began with the Keto Zone diet (see appendix F), which is an eating plan I outline in one of my previous books, but he relaxed it a bit. For him, he was the one who had let his body slide to where it was, and he wanted to be the one to get back to where he knew it should be. He basically used the Keto Zone as an outline as he went about his day. On the Keto Zone diet:

- Carbs are supposed to be 15 percent of the daily intake (mostly from salads, vegetables, spices, and herbs), but Terrance ate a few more carbs, trying to not miss the time around the table with his wife and young son.

- Fat is supposed to be 70 percent of daily intake (from modest amounts of fish oil, avocado oil, olive oil, seeds, nuts, and grass-fed butter), and he almost hit that amount with his food choices.

- As for proteins, which are to be 15 percent of daily intake (from whole pastured eggs, wild fish, and grass-fed meats), he upped the normal 1 g of protein per 1 kg of body weight a bit more.

For drinks he chose water, coffee, tea, and low-sugar almond or coconut milk. He cut out all sodas, sports drinks, and alcohol (except for a small glass of wine when company came over). Alkaline water was his mainstay, with two cups of coffee spaced throughout the morning and early afternoon.

For snacks he especially loved celery with cream cheese or peanut butter, but he also ate nuts (macadamia, pecans, almonds, walnuts, and sunflower seeds) during the day at work. He always avoided desserts, unless it was a birthday or special occasion, and then would only eat a few bites and stop.

He also took several supplements, such as a multivitamin, fish oil, vitamin D_3, and a probiotic. He also took DIM, which increases free testosterone levels (see appendix F). Changing his diet meant creating new habits, but he was motivated. He also found an exercise program that fit his schedule and met his testosterone-boosting needs. It was pretty simple:

- lifting weights (barbells) for about fifteen minutes each evening, with two-minute sprints on his stationary bicycle between weight sets

- going for walks with his family as many evenings as possible

As for "chilling" his body to reduce the stress he knew he lived under, he began to listen to the Bible on CD and soothing Christian music instead of talk radio while in the car to and from work. Getting his mind off the commute and relaxing his mind and body was the goal. He also upped his sleep to seven to eight hours each night. He had no caffeine late at night and certainly didn't binge-watch TV shows. And he made sure he spent ten to twenty minutes each morning over a cup of coffee reading his Bible, meditating on a verse, or praying.

IT'S A FACT

Your body produces the majority of testosterone while you are sleeping.[3] Getting a good night's sleep is indeed your needed "beauty rest."

The combined mental relaxation in the car and increased sleep would boost his adrenal gland reserve by decreasing the amount of cortisol his body had been producing while under extreme, nonstop stress. And since cortisol lowers testosterone levels, fixing this one area would have a compound beneficial effect on his body.

After three months he noticed quite a few changes. His waistline was already shrinking, he saw more muscle definition in his arms, and he felt more relaxed within himself and more focused at work. At the six-month mark he came to my office for a checkup. We ran his blood work, and I knew his numbers across the board would be better, even his cholesterol, though that wasn't our focus. He looked better, was noticeably stronger, and was proud of the fact that he had shed twenty-four pounds.

"I've got a few pounds to go, probably ten to twenty, but I know I'm making progress," he stated. "But the biggest change is probably in my head. I feel more alert, more rested, and more like my normal self. I like what I'm doing."

He explained his exercise program and how he used his drive time to both fuel and calm his body. As for food, he gave me a quick rundown of his favorite breakfasts, lunches, and dinners. It was basically the Keto Zone diet. This was his new healthy foundation, and after six months his numbers were pretty impressive.

YOUR FOUNDATION FOR HORMONE HEALTH

At thirty-five Terrance was not yet sick, but he knew what fate awaited him if he continued down the road he was on. Obesity, prediabetes, type 2 diabetes, and heart disease were no doubt close by, along with the many other illnesses associated with those diseases. He had several friends just a few years older than him who were already on medications, and their lives were not examples he wanted to aspire to.

"It is lethargic living," he stressed. "I refuse to let my body go that way. My wife and son deserve a healthy me, as do I." I agreed, but it was a decision that he had made himself, and he had been the one to make it happen. Nobody could do it for him. Terrance had laid a foundation for his future health that would pay him dividends for his entire life.

So what were his new hormone numbers after six months of eating differently, exercising, and creating good all-around lifestyle habits? We were both impressed:

Total T: 625 ng/dL

Free T3: 3.5 pg/mL

His numbers were now that of a healthy thirty-five-year-old! Remember, the range for total T in men is 264–916 ng/dL. At 625 ng/dL, Terrance was over the middle, and that is pretty good. And his free T3 (with the normal range being 2.0–4.4 pg/mL and the optimal range being 3.5–4.4 pg/mL) at 3.5 pg/mL moved from the low end of normal to the low end of the optimal range. Both of these numbers could be even higher, but they were great considering where he had been. I also checked his cholesterol numbers, along with other numbers from his blood work, and he was looking good overall.

Whether you are male or female, I recommend a diet very similar to what Terrance chose. Women can eat a little less protein than men, but overall the Keto Zone diet is one of the best lifestyle diets you can be on because it is anti-inflammatory and burns fat. Did you notice how few carbs are included in the Keto Zone diet from breads, bagels, cereals, and such? The key factor is lowering inflammation by choosing anti-inflammatory foods and lowering sugars, carbohydrates, and starches dramatically.

You may be wondering, "Can I boost all my different hormones by improving my lifestyle (changing my diet, exercising, taking supplements, having less stress, getting more sleep, and so on)?" The answer is a resounding *yes*! But let me ask you a question: How much boosting of your hormones do you need?

If you, like Terrance, want to get your body back in shape and increase your hormone levels, then doing what he did will probably be sufficient to meet your hormone needs, and the supplements in appendix F will probably help. However, that may not be everything your body requires. Perhaps your needs are different. Maybe you are more like these patients:

Ann, age thirty-one, cannot get pregnant, probably because her hormones are out of whack.

Carl, age sixty-two, cannot lower his cholesterol no matter what he eats or how he exercises and does not want to take cholesterol-lowering medications.

Patty, age seventy-five, has not had a sexual climax in more than twenty years.

Robert, age fifty-six, had his father die from Alzheimer's and doesn't want the same fate.

Kara, age forty-four, had a full hysterectomy and cannot seem to control her weight.

James, age seventy-two, is losing muscle fast and cannot stop the creep toward feebleness and frailty (sarcopenia).

Mindy, age sixty-eight, has osteoporosis and knows that if she falls and breaks a bone, she will probably eventually end up in a nursing home.

Janice, age fifty-seven, is starting to experience symptoms of arthritis in her hands, but she is a painter and cannot afford to lose her source of income.

Louise, age sixty-one, feels as if she is finding a new wrinkle on her face, neck, or arms every time she looks in the mirror.

Kristen, age twenty-nine, suffers from fibromyalgia.

The diet, exercise program, and less-stressful living will probably not increase these patients' hormone levels enough to counter the symptoms they suffer from. Yes, the Keto Zone diet is a great place to start. I think it is the foundation for everyone who wants to improve his or her hormone levels, but it may not be enough to get you where you want to go Why?

This is something everyone must understand: increasing your hormone levels through diet, exercise, supplements, and nutrition is possible to a certain degree, but to optimize your hormone levels, you usually need bioidentical hormone replacement therapy unless you are less than forty years of age like Terrance. Or look at it another way.

IT'S A FACT

The only way you are going to prevent feebleness and frailty
with aging is by optimizing your hormones.

If you need to stop sickness and disease or need to rebuild, restore, or regrow what has been lost, you need to optimize your hormone levels. Every one of these patients listed previously found help, answers, and freedom from symptoms when he or she optimized hormones. It was incredible to see!

Food and fitness are not strong enough to push back the aging process, to overcome the endocrine disruptors we all face in life, or to combat many of the diseases out there. Only hormones possess that power. That means the only way you are going to *optimize* your hormones (to the levels you had when you were in your twenties) is with bioidentical hormone replacement therapy.

And only when your hormones are optimized do you get all the incredible health benefits that come with it. These patients still had their symptoms when we had balanced their hormones, but as we kept raising their hormone levels to a high normal or optimal level, the symptoms began to subside. After several months at the optimized level, along with the healthy Keto Zone foundational diet, usually most of the symptoms were gone. And sometimes every single one of those uncomfortable, debilitating, embarrassing, hated symptoms was gone!

You know what your health needs are, but if you are looking for help, answers, and freedom from your symptoms, then I strongly suggest that you look at optimizing your hormones. One more thing you need to understand: There is nothing wrong with needing hormone replacement therapy. There is also no "grin and bear it" prize in life.

And it isn't that you are somehow cheating. After all, your body probably had optimized hormones when you were in your twenties, and we are only trying to get you back to that point.

When your hormone levels are optimized and most of your symptoms have fallen away, you will know exactly what I'm talking about. Living with optimized hormones is the best way to live!

CHAPTER 6

AN EXAMPLE OF HOW HORMONE THERAPY CAN WORK FOR YOU

T'S BEEN ABOUT twenty years," Elaine, who was seventy years old, said. "I started to notice the loss of muscle before I turned fifty, but it has only sped up since then."

"Was that the only issue?" I asked.

"Oh no," she responded. "I gradually started having less muscle in my arms and legs and more fat in its place. Then it was fatigue, joint pain, sleep issues, and osteoporosis."

Elaine's daughter was with us at the doctor visit. She added, "Also, the doctor my mom had before she moved down here to be near us and the grandkids said that she has mild type 2 diabetes."

I flipped through her charts. "And from the look of your reports, they stopped giving you synthetic thyroid [Synthroid] several years ago but still have you on antidepressants and sleeping meds."

"Yes, I was supposed to talk to my doctor about diabetes, but with the move and everything, I haven't done that yet," Elaine added. As she talked, I was reminded of what renowned OB-GYN physician Gary Donovitz says about aging.

> To age, deteriorate, lose strength, energy, and sexual function and feel lousy is commonly treated by physicians with a pat on the back and an antidepressant—which is not what patients want or need.[1]

To his list I would add other common ailments, such as pain, inflammation, depression, brain fog, weight gain, muscle and bone loss, and poor memory. But he is right; patients need and want more than a pat on the back. They deserve more, and that includes help in the form of real answers.

"Elaine, it sounds like you have been suffering from sarcopenia these past twenty years," I noted. "Sarcopenia is the wasting away of muscle that is replaced with fatty tissue, and it only increases as we age. That would certainly explain some of your symptoms."

They both nodded their heads in agreement.

"But I also have some good news for you."

The look on Elaine's daughter's face was one of hope. Elaine's was more of a desperation look, but either way, they wanted answers. I could read that in their expressions.

"Your symptoms, from sarcopenia to osteoporosis and from joint pain to type 2 diabetes, are a clear indicator that your hormone levels are extremely low," I explained.

"But my TSH level is still in normal range," Elaine interjected.

"It might be, but the TSH is not the best indicator of your active thyroid hormone levels," I pointed out.

"And the good news?" Elaine's daughter asked.

"We can usually treat most of her symptoms with bioidentical hormone replacement therapy," I answered. "When we optimize your hormone levels, we will not only treat those symptoms; I would not be surprised if we roll back most of those symptoms and even prevent future illness."

They both smiled. Elaine let out a big breath and then said, "When can we start? I have finally moved near my grandbabies, and I want to enjoy them for many years to come."

BEATING ILLNESS WITH HORMONE THERAPY

Very few people are told that the risk of heart disease, type 2 diabetes, Alzheimer's, breast cancer, prostate cancer, and osteoporosis decreases with hormone replacement therapy.[2] But it does! I have found in my practice that many diseases are stopped completely and the symptoms are reversed when we optimize our hormone levels. As for Elaine's osteoporosis, bone can regrow at around 8 percent per year when hormones are optimized, and I have experienced that with several patients. How often do osteoporosis sufferers hear that good bit of news?

IT'S A FACT

As of 2017, according to the Arthritis Foundation, more than one in two men and more than two in three women over age sixty-five may have arthritis.[3]

With Elaine, it was her sarcopenia that was causing her the greatest number of issues. Get that taken care of, and her host of other ailments would also fade away. Everyone has heard about osteoporosis and how the loss of bone mass is debilitating. It is something people, especially women, try to avoid as they age. Hardly anyone talks about sarcopenia, yet it affects millions of people.[4]

What causes sarcopenia? It is the result of anabolic hormones being low or low normal for a long time, along with several other issues, including:

- lack of digestive enzymes and/or HCL
- lack of protein
- lack of exercise
- nutritional imbalances
- stress
- inflammation[5]

The main hormone being "out of sync" is testosterone. It is, as you know, the hormone most responsible for muscle growth.

Men gradually start losing testosterone in their thirties, but women begin to lose testosterone in their twenties! Both men and women need testosterone because when testosterone levels go low, people are at greater risk of:

- muscle loss (sarcopenia)
- bone loss (osteoporosis)
- depression
- lack of energy
- lack of mental clarity
- weight gain (especially around the belly)

- difficulty losing weight
- anxiety
- irritability
- heart disease
- type 2 diabetes
- low sex drive
- prostate cancer and ED for men
- Alzheimer's
- Parkinson's
- dementia

SARCOPENIA EVENTUALLY AFFECTS US ALL

Many of these symptoms on the list accurately described Elaine, but she is certainly not alone. That is because between ages thirty and sixty most people will likely gain about a pound of fat a year and lose about a half a pound of muscle a year. Put another way, over a thirty-year time span the change in body composition of the average adult equals fifteen pounds of muscle loss and thirty pounds of fat gain.[6]

IT'S A FACT

Nursing homes are holding tanks for people. I believe sarcopenia is one of the main reasons we end up there. It's usually from low testosterone, which is preventable and treatable.

That means most people, because they are "average," are going to be looking at sarcopenia in their future. Fortunately for them it doesn't usually affect them in their fifties, as it did Elaine. Rather, it most often hits when they are in their seventies, especially around age seventy-five.

You see it all the time. People suffering from sarcopenia are hunched over, have little muscle, are frail, are feeble, have fat instead of muscle, have virtually no leg muscles, and have their skin hanging from their bone. That is sarcopenia!

But according to the CDC, the average person in the United States can expect to live to 78.8 years.[7] And with the focus on osteoporosis, which is directly related to sarcopenia, very few people are diagnosed well enough in advance to ward off the sarcopenia before it takes a heavy toll.

If you are over age forty, you should get an annual blood test to make sure your hormone levels are where you want them to be. When you do, ask that they test:

- total testosterone
- free testosterone
- TSH
- free T3
- TPO
- reverse T3 (rT3)
- estradiol
- progesterone (for women)
- follicle-stimulating hormone (FSH, for women)

Usually it is low testosterone levels that bring about sarcopenia and osteoporosis in my patients. Sarcopenia and osteoporosis are related conditions, which means it's common for one condition to accompany or follow the other.[8]

According to the Administration on Aging, the US population age sixty-five and older (currently about forty-nine million people) is expected to grow past ninety-eight million by 2060.[9] With that warning of sarcopenia in mind, consider:

Back in 2000, a third of the 1.5 million people admitted to long-term health care facilities were placed there because they weren't able to perform daily living activities.[10]

It is believed that sarcopenia affects 5–13 percent of people age sixty to seventy and 11–50 percent of individuals eighty and over.[11] Since this disease is rarely recognized by most doctors, I feel these numbers are much higher.

Older people who have sarcopenia have a greater risk of becoming disabled—1.5 to 4.6 times higher—than those who don't suffer from sarcopenia.[12]

Skeletal muscle mass is estimated to decrease 35–40 percent between the ages of twenty and eighty for both men and women.[13]

People can slow the rate of muscle loss and weakening through diet and exercise, but even senior adults who are active will experience a decrease in muscle function.[14]

That is pretty scary, especially since we all want to live to a nice old age!

THE COSTLY EFFECTS OF SARCOPENIA

What adds another layer of worry to the mix is the cost of sarcopenia. In 2000 it was estimated that US health care costs associated with sarcopenia were around $20 billion.[15] They even put a personal price tag on that, estimating it to be about $900 per person per year.[16]

The disease itself is not the only cost. Each year in the United States, more than $26 billion is spent to provide added care for people who can no longer live independently.[17] And as you would expect, people with troubles caused by sarcopenia will naturally have more doctor visits and fill more prescriptions than those without those problems, which adds even more expense to the health care system.[18]

IT'S A FACT

Optimized hormones often stop or prevent many of the diseases that plague the elderly, including sarcopenia, osteoporosis, and dementia.

The loss of muscle is one of the worst things that can happen to our bodies. Muscle is one of the best indicators of health and serves as a barrier against weight gain, illness, diabetes, cancers, memory-related illnesses, and much more. Sarcopenia and its muscle-wasting effects open the door directly to insulin resistance, type 2 diabetes, and obesity.[19] And we have already discussed the multitude of diseases that follow obesity around.

It is estimated that by 2050 one in three people will have type 2 diabetes, and the disease's prevalence could double or even triple from 2010 to 2050![20] The annual cost of diabetes was $174 billion in 2010.[21]

Is all of this sickness and crazy expense directly the result of sarcopenia? No, but sarcopenia does play a part. You see, sarcopenia is itself just a symptom, usually a symptom of long-term low testosterone levels. Is testosterone to blame? No, because you cannot blame the absence of something for causing anything. However, when low testosterone is reversed and optimized:

- bone mass regrows, which helps stop and reverse osteoporosis
- muscles regrow, which helps stop and reverse sarcopenia
- bigger muscles improve insulin resistance, which helps stop and sometimes reverse type 2 diabetes
- weight is usually controlled, which helps stop belly fat and obesity
- a positive outlook is maintained, which helps stop depression
- the heart is strengthened, and testosterone usually helps lower bad (LDL) cholesterol
- energy levels are usually boosted, which helps stop fatigue
- muscle and bone pains are usually relieved, which usually helps stop or lessen muscle and joint inflammation
- the brain is protected, which helps prevent dementia

Countless symptoms, sicknesses, and diseases seep into your aging body as your hormone levels get lower and lower. Even having enough testosterone to be "in range" is not enough to combat many of these ailments. Only by optimizing your testosterone levels does your body have the ability to regain what it needs for healthy living.

LOOKING FOR GOOD RESULTS

When Elaine first came, her numbers were pretty low, just as you would expect with someone who battled sarcopenia, osteoporosis, and other ailments. Her testosterone number was a mere 12 ng/dL.

IT'S A FACT

Muscle-building exercises (without using actual weights) can also include push-ups, planks, sit-ups, squats, calf raises, running, and walking.

Less than six months later, after we optimized her testosterone levels, that number was 94 ng/dL. Now, these numbers won't mean much until you lay them beside the "in range" numbers and see just where she was.

The ranges vary, but 15–70 ng/dL is pretty common for testosterone levels with a woman her age. At 12 ng/dL she was virtually out of testosterone! My guess was that she had been running on empty for years! When we boosted her numbers up to 94 ng/dL, her tank was full, and that made all the difference. In short it looked like this:

starting point: 12 ng/dL (incredibly low)

normal range: 15–70 ng/dL (for most people)

almost six months later: 94 ng/dL (optimized) (Note: People with osteoporosis and sarcopenia need slightly higher testosterone levels to reverse osteoporosis and sarcopenia.)

In addition to optimizing her testosterone hormone levels, she also took other steps that are necessary to stop, remedy, and help prevent sarcopenia, which included:

Muscle-building exercises: Strength training (resistance training) uses weights or machines and progressively increases resistance against your muscles. This increases muscle mass, which protects against sarcopenia and even plays a part in reversing the negative effects of sarcopenia.[22] Strength training greatly improves your overall fitness, mobility, and bone health.[23]

Enzymes to help digestion: People over age seventy-five often need enzymes to help them digest their foods adequately, especially proteins. Hydrochloric acid with pepsin is also helpful. Lowering stress and increasing activity also helps aid proper digestion.

Lowering inflammation: This is often caused by medications, chronic infections, and inflammatory foods, as well as excessive stress. Elaine's lifestyle, including her medications and lack of exercise, were adding to the problem. Getting on an anti-inflammatory diet such as the Keto Zone diet (see appendix F) can significantly decrease inflammation.

People who suffer from sarcopenia also often have other low hormone levels, including human growth hormone (HGH) and dehydroepiandrosterone (DHEA).[24] We included these with Elaine's hormone replacement therapy and optimized both levels. Thankfully, regardless of age, when we optimize hormone levels and add proper exercise with the necessary nutritional supplements, our bodies can recover! Even as devastating as sarcopenia is, it can be reversed.

With Elaine, not only did her sarcopenia (and all her related symptoms) stop and begin to fade away, so did her osteoporosis. It reversed course without meds for osteoporosis. Her aches and pains disappeared as well, and she got off her antidepressant medication. These days she enjoys swimming laps at her condo pool and playing with her grandchildren. She is independent and drives her own car, and as far as I am concerned, she can keep this up for years and years to come.

Elaine's story hits pretty close to home for me. My mom is in her eighties, and she wants to be able to stay in her own home and live life to the fullest. The best thing I can do to make sure that happens is to optimize her hormones and encourage her to take the necessary supplements, increase her exercise regimen, and follow the Keto Zone diet.

My mom also has type 2 diabetes and has had it for many years, but by optimizing her hormone levels, we improved her insulin resistance considerably. But even bigger, we are reversing her osteoporosis. She has gained back some muscle mass, and all of it combined is helping prevent sarcopenia. Optimizing hormone levels truly works wonders!

Just One Disease of Many

Sarcopenia is just an example. It is one disease of many that are increasing in number today, such as heart disease, high cholesterol, obesity, fibromyalgia, type 2 diabetes, osteoporosis, Alzheimer's, Parkinson's, dementia, lupus, breast cancer, and many more. To me the connection is obvious: across the board disease rates are increasing, and our hormone levels are decreasing.

Sarcopenia is one of the many diseases that everyone would like to avoid. It is also a disease that optimized hormone levels can stop and reverse, and the body can be restored. With all the many symptoms and diseases out there, the answer is still the same: optimizing your hormone levels.

It feels good to expect great results, doesn't it?

CHAPTER 7

QUESTIONS ANSWERED ABOUT YOUR HORMONE THERAPY

HIS ARMS WERE bulging with muscles. They were Joe's pride and joy. Approaching sixty years of age, he could easily outperform most of the other policemen in his department. He wasn't an outright bodybuilder, but he did everything he could to boost his testosterone levels, including getting shots from another doctor across town.

"But doc, I've got a few symptoms I'm wondering if you can help me with," he said the first afternoon he came by my office. I was wondering what his symptoms might be. He looked in tip-top shape. "I really don't want to talk about this, but my wife said I should," he began. "Well, here it is: I can't seem to keep an erection. In fact, I'm not really interested in sex at all. What is happening to me? Am I doing something wrong?"

He was very knowledgeable about his health and hormone levels, so I asked, "What are your testosterone numbers? And free T numbers?"

"My testosterone is just past 2000, and my free T is at 400," he stated matter-of-factly.

I've heard of bodybuilders with testosterone levels around 2500 and free T over 500. I would not recommend his numbers to people, but he was seeing another doctor who was prescribing the testosterone. "What about your estradiol numbers?" I asked.

"My what?" he replied. "That's an estrogen, isn't it? I don't think I have a problem with that."

"We need to look at your estradiol numbers because your symptoms match those of someone with elevated estradiol hormone levels," I explained. "Just by chance, do you find yourself watching a movie

67

or reading a book and crying? You know, the old 'it's dusty in here' thing?"

He laughed, "Actually, I have been feeling more sentimental and emotional than normal. I thought it was kinda weird."

JOE'S NUMBERS

Testosterone range for men over eighteen years of age: 264–916 ng/dL

Optimized testosterone levels should be: 800–1100 ng/dL

Joe's testosterone levels: 2046 ng/dL

Free T range for men ages eighteen to seventy: 46–224 pg/mL

Optimized free T levels should be: 150–224 pg/mL

Joe's free T levels: 400 pg/mL

Estradiol range for men over eighteen years of age: 20–70 pg/mL

Optimized estradiol levels should be: 20–50 pg/mL

Joe's estradiol levels: 140 pg/mL

We ran his blood work, and a week later I had him stop by for a quick chat. "You ready for this?" I began with a smile, holding up his paperwork.

"Sure. I can take it," he answered.

"OK, to put it bluntly, you have the estrogen levels, estradiol in particular, of a young woman." I paused, letting those words sink in. "Your estradiol number is 140 pg/mL, and it should be between 20 and 70 pg/mL. I recommend in the 20–50 pg/mL range."

"What does that mean, and what can I do to fix it?" he asked.

We took a few minutes, and I discussed how men begin to convert more and more testosterone to estradiol as they age due to increased activity of the aromatase enzyme. This is evidenced in the usual fat in the belly, breasts, back, chest, and sides. In Joe's case his excessive amount of testosterone was converting to more estradiol than he was normally used to.

"Can I do anything about it?" he repeated, a hint of worry in his voice.

"Yes, this is actually pretty easy to fix," I reassured him.

He needed to start taking diindolylmethane (DIM), a natural supplement made from broccoli that acts as a natural aromatase inhibitor (reduces estrogen conversion). I suggested he take 150 mg of DIM twice a day to lower his estradiol to an acceptable range. That usually works for most men trying to lower their estrogen levels.

The good thing about DIM is that it will not push estrogen levels too low. Some aromatase inhibitors, such as Arimidex, can lower estrogen levels to unhealthy levels, but DIM does not. The fact is, we all need our estrogen, both men and women, and DIM lowers estrogen levels in men without wiping estrogen out completely. (See appendix F.)

Joe started taking 150 mg of DIM, once after breakfast and once after dinner, and when we checked his estradiol level just six weeks later, it was 64 pg/mL. That was a huge drop down from 140 pg/mL! I also had Joe lower his testosterone dosage to half of what he was taking. And his symptoms?

"Gone—completely gone!" he said with a hearty laugh.

QUESTIONS AND MORE QUESTIONS

Hormones have been caught in a whirlpool of confusion for more than a century. It only makes sense then that questions swirl when we start using hormone replacement therapy to address very real symptoms, sicknesses, and diseases. All questions are important because nobody wants to do anything blindly, especially when it comes to good health and enjoying life. The following are some of the most common questions that surround hormone replacement therapy.

Q: WHAT ARE HORMONES?

Hormones are often described as messengers that carry messages from one cell to another. These messages tell cells what to do. Another way to look at it is to imagine hormones as the letters of this sentence. Each letter goes in the right order to convey a thought. Scramble the order, remove a few letters, or send all the letters at the same time, and you have chaos. It's a mess, utterly worthless, but at least the letters can't physically hurt you! At the cellular level when the messenger hormones are negatively impacted, you have very real damage in the form of symptoms, sickness, chronic illness, and eventually death.

Q: WHY DO WE NEED HORMONE THERAPY?

Chapter 4 answers this question more comprehensively, but here is the answer in a nutshell. Due to health, diet, lifestyle choices—what we touch, what we eat, medications we take, deficiencies in our diet, stress—and the aging process itself, our hormone levels eventually become so low that we usually develop debilitating symptoms, illnesses, and diseases. Low hormone levels cause fatigue and many other symptoms, which often means we are inviting a multitude of chronic diseases into our lives, and therefore, we need hormone replacement therapy.

Q: DO I NEED HORMONE THERAPY?

At the individual level your own needs are different from those of someone else, those of your parents, siblings, children, and other family members. Everyone is different. Your body needs adequate or optimized hormone levels to prevent many diseases, but if you have developed symptoms that are negatively impacting your life, or you are trying to avoid disease later in life, then hormone therapy is a great answer.

Q: IS HORMONE THERAPY HEALTHY?

Bioidentical hormones are healthy and actually good for you! For example, bioidentical progesterone may reduce cancer risk,[1] treats PMS, and helps women sleep. Bioidentical estrogen treats the effects of aging and stress, menopause symptoms, and atrophic vaginitis and prevents osteoporosis. Bioidentical testosterone helps strengthen the body from the effects of age and stress; maintains muscle, bone, and mental focus; protects the heart; improves cholesterol levels; delays diabetes; and maintains normal sexual function.[2] Sign me up!

Q: ARE ALL HORMONES CREATED EQUAL?

No! All the big hormone scares, hoaxes, myths, and flawed studies have been based on the bad side effects of synthetic hormones. You would be surprised at the faulty logic that has confused the world about hormones. Imagine saying the inability to digest a plastic grape from the display cabinet is sufficient reason to stop eating fresh grapes! Simply stated, synthetic hormones are not the same as bioidentical hormones. Remember, numerous studies have found that synthetic progestin causes breast cancer, while the bioidentical progesterone actually prevents breast cancer. The differences between synthetic and bioidentical hormones are astounding.

Q: IS A PRESCRIPTION REQUIRED?

Yes, you need a prescription to get bioidentical hormone therapy. The other parts, such as supplements and vitamins, are available at any health food store. See appendix F for supplements to support hormone health.

Q: WHAT DOES IT COST?

It depends on the type of hormone replacement therapy you choose to do and the frequency of your dosage. If you need a higher dose more often, the price will be more. Prices vary, but patients can usually expect to pay from $50 to $120 a month for bioidentical hormone therapy. Considering the health savings alone, this will pay you great dividends. Insurance companies will often cover some of the expense. Compounding pharmacies are usually able to compound testosterone cream much cheaper than AndroGel, which is the testosterone gel that is prescribed by most physicians.

Q: WHAT ARE THE DIFFERENT APPLICATION METHODS OF HORMONE THERAPY?

There are many different ways to get hormones into your body. Orally (taking pills) is the worst way, as it may harm the liver, so that is not an option. Other options (which I'll discuss further in later chapters) include:

- shots (usually with a very small needle injected into your thigh or buttock)
- pellets (A pellet the size of a grain of rice is inserted usually painlessly into your hip area.)
- patches (These go on your arms or legs, like bandages.)
- sublingual tablets (These dissolve under your tongue and rarely stress the liver.)
- creams and gels (applied to hairless areas on your body—e.g., back of the knee or shoulder)

Currently shots and pellets are usually the best methods to boost hormones into the optimal range. There is a new cream base (called Atrevis base) that delivers testosterone through the skin by using three naturally derived permeation enhancers. Studies show that Atrevis can deliver almost three times as much testosterone through the skin as other bases.[3] This makes it possible to obtain optimal levels formerly only achieved with pellets and shots.

Q: HOW OFTEN DO I NEED IT?

The frequency of application depends on your needs and the method you choose. Here are common application rates:

- Shots can range from every other day to once or twice a week.
- Pellets can be taken once every three to four months for women or once every five to six months for men.
- Creams and gels can be used once a day.

Q: WHERE DO I FIND A BIOIDENTICAL HORMONE REPLACEMENT DOCTOR?

There are online directories of doctors who practice bioidentical hormone replacement therapy. (You can find a list of helpful websites in appendix F.) There are probably many doctors in your local area who use bioidentical hormone replacement therapy with their patients. Ask around, look online for local doctors, and ask them if they use bioidentical hormones in their treatment. You may have to drive a little further than you would normally go for your primary doctor, but it will be worth it. Also, do not feel pressured to use only one form of treatment. Find out all the facts, and choose the method that is best for you.

Q: WHY OPTIMIZE INSTEAD OF BALANCE HORMONES?

Balanced hormones are certainly better than hormones out of balance, but many symptoms usually persist even after you have balanced your hormone levels. However, when you optimize your hormone levels, pushing them to the level they were at when you were in your twenties, symptoms usually disappear and diseases are often stopped, reversed, and prevented. Make sure your bioidentical hormone replacement doctor is willing to optimize rather than just balance your hormone levels. Consider optimizing all your hormones. You should have your hormones that were low rechecked after six to eight weeks of hormone therapy and then every three to six months thereafter.

Q: MY HORMONES ARE "IN RANGE," BUT MY SYMPTOMS WON'T GO AWAY. WHAT DO I DO?

You need to boost your hormone levels higher, ideally into the optimized range. This will usually start to relieve your symptoms and eventually may remove them entirely. Because most doctors do not treat hormone issues at all, or they wait until your hormone levels are lower than what is considered the "normal" range (which means you are most likely very sick), you have to keep looking until you find a doctor who will address your symptoms with bioidentical hormone replacement therapy.

Q: CAN I BOOST MY HORMONES NATURALLY?

Bioidentical hormones are natural, but if by "natural" you mean boosting your hormone levels through diet, nutrition, supplements, exercise, sleep, and less stress, then you absolutely can. Such a foundation to healthy living will usually increase your hormone levels across the board. (See chapter 5.) The more you take care of yourself, the better. But as we've discussed, if you cannot raise your hormone levels higher (after you've maxed a healthy diet and lifestyle and supplements), or you want to optimize your hormone levels for health reasons, then hormone therapy is the only way to accomplish that. (See appendix F for supplements that boost hormone levels.)

Q: IS NUTRITION STRONG ENOUGH TO BALANCE HORMONES?

Yes, with careful diet and nutrition, including quite a few supplements, it is certainly possible to balance most hormone levels for a time, but eventually with age hormone levels will decline. For years I helped patients balance their hormones, but it can be pricey and taking ten to fifteen supplements is too much for many people. But do you want to balance or optimize your hormones? If you want to optimize your hormone levels, then nutrition is not usually strong enough. There is great power in hormones. It is my firm belief that you need bioidentical hormone therapy to optimize hormone levels. Needless to say, part of optimizing your hormones includes a good diet, nutrition, exercise, sleep, good water, and less stress. (These are six of the seven pillars in my book *The Seven Pillars of Health*.) It all works together.

Q: DO I HAVE TO GO GLUTEN-FREE?

Gluten is a protein that may inflame the thyroid and the GI tract. With most patients who are working hard to optimize their hormone levels, gluten has to go. For most Hashimoto's patients, they definitely need to give up gluten. So ask yourself, "Am I willing to give up donuts, pretzels, bagels, bread, crackers, chips, pasta, and more to get my hormones in order?" If not, then you can certainly *balance* your hormone levels. But hormone *optimization* may require that you go gluten-free.

Q: WHAT ARE "SEX HORMONES"?

You have many hormones, but only three—testosterone, estrogen, and progesterone—are considered "sex hormones," because they are responsible for sexual development and fertility. These hormones also provide a long list of other benefits, such as weight loss, improved eyesight, muscle growth, bone strengthening, improved mood, and better sleep. Not all hormones are sex hormones, and clearly even those that are sex hormones are not all about sex.

IT'S A FACT

It is estimated that stress-related problems account for as much as 90 percent of all doctor visits.[4]

Q: DOES STRESS REALLY AFFECT HORMONE LEVELS?

Yes, your hormones become imbalanced if you are under stress. When the stress does not stop, such as chronic worry, anxiety, illness, pain, depression, fibromyalgia, and so on, the continued cortisol secretion lowers your other hormones, including sex hormones and thyroid hormones. Lowered hormone levels naturally raise your risk for disease, preceded by countless dreadful symptoms. Excessive or long-term stress, such as a chronic illness, anxiety, depression, chronic pain, a bad marriage, or a stressful job or daily commute, can cause your cortisol levels to remain elevated day after day, year after year. When this happens, usually the production of other hormones is put on the back burner, and this in turn leads to more and more hormone imbalances and deficiencies. In women I have found that testosterone, progesterone, and thyroid are especially affected by long-term stress.

Q: IS IT POSSIBLE MY PRESCRIPTIONS ARE MESSING WITH MY HORMONE LEVELS?

Absolutely! It's not only possible; it's probable. The drugs that doctors prescribe for our aches, depression, high cholesterol, weight gain, anxiety, insomnia, hot flashes, stress, and so on will usually not fix the core issue of low hormone levels. What's worse, the medications they prescribe may lower your hormone levels even more. When your hormone levels are optimized, many prescribed medications may no longer be necessary.

Q: ARE THERE SIDE EFFECTS FROM BIOIDENTICAL HORMONE THERAPY?

There can be, but they are easily treatable. (That is not true for synthetic hormones, as many studies have shown how dangerous they are.) When you discuss your hormone replacement therapy plan with your doctor, you will also figure out the best method of application. At that point any side effects will be addressed, and you will know what you can do to avoid any discomfort. A side effect with bioidentical estrogen is vaginal bleeding or spotting and cramping, but this usually doesn't occur if taking an adequate dosage of micronized progesterone. Remember, bioidentical testosterone helps protect women from breast cancer. Bioidentical estrogen does not cause cancer but could fuel cancer. Before I place women on bioidentical estrogen, I have them do a mammogram to screen for breast cancer. If the patient has the BRCA1 or BRCA2 gene mutation, she should not be on any estrogen.

Q: WILL HORMONE REPLACEMENT THERAPY CAUSE CANCER, BLOOD CLOTS, BONE LOSS, OR STROKES?

These exact fears have proved to be true when using *synthetic* hormones. However, as I've stressed throughout this book, numerous studies have found *bioidentical* hormones—which are identical to the hormones that you produced in abundance when you were younger—to prevent cancer, reduce the risk of blood clots, stop bone loss, restore bone mass by more than 8 percent each year, improve blood flow, reduce blood pressure, grow muscle, and even lower cholesterol. One recent multiyear study showed that older men with low testosterone and preexisting coronary artery disease can reduce their risk of stroke, heart attack, and death with testosterone therapy.[5] I have found the same results apply to women.

Q: WILL OPTIMIZING MY HORMONES HELP ME OVERCOME OBESITY?

Yes, and it is easy to treat! Stats show about 40 percent of men (and I have found the same is true in women) are obese, and obesity increases our risks for heart disease, type 2 diabetes, Alzheimer's, dementia, strokes, erectile dysfunction, autoimmune disorders, arthritis, osteoporosis, sarcopenia, and many other diseases simply because the fatter people are, the sicker they usually get.[6] Testosterone levels are usually low or suboptimal in obese people, but I have found that by treating my obese patients with the Keto Zone diet (see appendix F) and exercise added to hormone optimization, metabolic rates improve dramatically. That means fat burns as a person sleeps. What is more, it saves money! Obese people spend over one hundred dollars per month more in medical costs than non-obese people.[7]

IT'S A FACT

Obesity is not the same as being overweight; obesity is having an unhealthy amount of body fat. Body mass index (BMI) is a person's weight (in kilograms) divided by his height (in meters) squared. A high BMI can indicate a high level of body fat, which is why BMI is a more accurate measure of obesity than weight. Adults with a BMI of 30 or higher are considered obese.[8] Many health organization websites have BMI calculators to help you do the math, such as https://www.nhlbi.nih.gov/health/educational/lose_wt/BMI/bmicalc.htm for adults and https://www.cdc.gov/healthyweight/bmi/calculator.html for children and teens.

Q: HOW CAN MEN KEEP THEIR ESTROGEN LEVELS FROM CREEPING UP AS THEY AGE?

Men should check their hormone levels (review Joe's story at the beginning of this chapter), especially their estrogen levels. They can get hormone replacement therapy if necessary, but usually 150 mg of diindolylmethane (DIM) twice a day will lower their estrogen levels. The DIM supplement is available at health food stores.

Q: SHOULD WOMEN WHO HAVE HAD BREAST CANCER AVOID HORMONE THERAPY?

The answer will vary according to doctors, but I may prescribe estriol vaginal cream (to protect them from atrophic vaginitis) and testosterone (which helps protect against cancer) for women in remission if their oncologist agrees to it. I do not recommend any estrogen or testosterone or progesterone if a woman has active breast cancer. Estriol is the weakest estrogen and has the least stimulating effect on the breast and uterus. Estriol has been used in Europe for many years and has been shown to not promote breast cancer and may in fact protect against it.[9] This has worked well with many women who have had breast cancer and are now in remission yet need the benefits that estriol cream and testosterone can bring to their bodies. I find that a testosterone pellet with an estrogen blocker (Arimidex) works well for most of my patients with a past history of breast cancer. If a person has breast cancer and wants either of the hormones, I have the patient get permission from her oncologist. Some will give permission; some won't. I also provide them with articles if they are interested.

Q: WILL HORMONE THERAPY MAKE MEN IMPOTENT?

Many prescribed medications cause impotence (erectile dysfunction), which I discuss elsewhere, by lowering already low testosterone levels. Taking testosterone will usually do the opposite and may completely eliminate erectile dysfunction issues. Optimized testosterone levels will usually increase energy levels, improve metabolism, burn fat, lower blood pressure, improve diabetes, and lift depression. No impotence there!

Q: IS THERE A CONNECTION BETWEEN PROSTATE CANCER AND LOW TESTOSTERONE?

Men with low testosterone levels (less than 250 ng/dL) are twice as likely to get prostate cancer than those who have normal testosterone levels.[10] Some say that low testosterone protects men from prostate cancer, but the exact opposite is true.[11] Higher testosterone levels are healthier for men, especially if they are worried about their prostate. Optimizing testosterone levels with bioidentical hormones will not cause prostate cancer. One of the most renowned urologists in the world, Dr. Abraham Morgentaler, agrees with this.[12]

Q: CAN HORMONE THERAPY PROTECT AGAINST ALZHEIMER'S, PARKINSON'S, OR DEMENTIA?

I believe that optimizing your hormone levels is the most effective way to protect against, treat, and sometimes even reverse memory-related diseases. The results in my patients have been astounding, though they naturally vary with each person. If you have these symptoms or diseases, or are trying to protect yourself from them, then I believe optimizing your hormones is the absolute best treatment plan.

Q: CAN HORMONE THERAPY LOWER CHOLESTEROL LEVELS?

Yes, optimizing testosterone, progesterone, thyroid, and estrogen hormone levels will usually lower bad cholesterol and raise good cholesterol. For years, it has been shown that healthy thyroid numbers lower total cholesterol.[13] Interestingly optimizing thyroid levels lowers cholesterol and decreases inflammation, doing precisely what statin drugs are supposed to do.[14]

Q: CAN HORMONE THERAPY HELP THOSE WITH PREDIABETES OR TYPE 2 DIABETES?

Prediabetics and type 2 diabetics usually have low hormone levels. In fact, men with type 2 diabetes are two times more likely to have low testosterone than their counterparts without diabetes.[15] Lowered hormone levels usually increase insulin resistance, which means the insulin is not working well to lower the blood sugar. That also means weight gain, which compounds the problems even further. People with prediabetes and type 2 diabetes are also on a lot of medications, and these medications usually lower hormone levels even further. I have found in treating my patients that optimizing hormone levels, along with the Keto Zone diet and exercise, has tremendous effects on weight loss, hemoglobin A1C levels, and correcting insulin resistance. Many times prediabetes and type 2 diabetes in my patients are completely reversed. It takes more effort to restore and reverse the damage if someone has had type 2 diabetes for more than fifteen years, but it can still be done.

Q: CAN HORMONE THERAPY HELP TREAT DEPRESSION?

Absolutely! The thyroid hormone T3 and testosterone are usually the answer. T3 is the most commonly used thyroid hormone in treating depression.[16] Speaking from experience, T3 gives my patients more energy, helps balance moods, boosts the immune system, improves skin, sharpens focus, speeds up metabolism, helps with weight loss, raises body temperature, lowers blood pressure and cholesterol, and much more. Testosterone also plays a part by helping boost dopamine levels, which helps incredibly when fighting depression. Depression can be a thing of the past!

Q: CAN HORMONE THERAPY HELP KEEP ME OUT OF A NURSING HOME?

The absolute best way to avoid being sent to a nursing home is to keep your muscles strong and your brain clear. Diseases such as sarcopenia, osteoporosis, and memory-related diseases are the quickest way to be admitted into a nursing home, but I have seen these health conditions minimized, and I believe in time we'll find they are being prevented in my patients who have chosen to optimize their hormone levels, especially testosterone.

Q: IS IT MORALLY WRONG TO GET HORMONE REPLACEMENT THERAPY?

No, there is nothing morally wrong with getting hormone replacement therapy. It is based on your body's need. When you were in your twenties, you had hormone levels that are much higher than they are today. Due to many factors, such as age, stress, hormone disruptors, and sickness, your hormone levels are probably much lower than they once were. We are only raising your hormone levels to what they once were. That is all.

Bioidentical hormone replacement therapy may be precisely what your body needs.

If you are ready, let's begin!

PART III
MAKING A GREAT LIFE WITH HORMONE THERAPY

PART 3 IS about how low or suboptimal levels of specific hormones affect your body and send you to the doctor, who usually prescribes medications that patch your symptoms rather than fixing the root problem. You will also discover how to stop the symptoms and many times reverse the disease when you optimize your hormone levels!

CHAPTER 8

THYROID TO REBOOT YOUR METABOLISM

J UNE DESCRIBED HERSELF as barely functioning with severe fatigue, depression, brain fog, and perpetual cold hands and cold feet. She came to my office with so many thyroid symptoms that it was like a jigsaw puzzle trying to piece it all together.

Thankfully she was willing to do whatever it took to regain her health. The sad news was that she had been battling these symptoms for many years, all while raising a family and helping her husband run a business.

To say she pressed through incredible health roadblocks would be putting it mildly. If people were awarded medals for living life despite their seemingly impossible situations, she would have been at the top of the podium. Instead of boring you with her symptoms, I will encourage you with her final results. Today she is a new woman:

- Her brain fog has lifted.
- Her aches and pains are a thing of the past.
- Her hair is thick again.
- Many of her wrinkles disappeared as her skin regained a more youthful look.
- She is full of energy, no longer crashing in the middle of the afternoon or after dinner.
- She no longer needs to take antidepressants.
- Her cold hands and cold feet became warm again.
- Her frequent migraines went away.
- She lost twenty pounds because she had energy and started walking, biking, and going to the gym.

Her treatment included natural desiccated thyroid (NDT), along with a few other over-the-counter supplements. She took the prescribed thyroid twice a day, once before breakfast on an empty stomach and another in the early afternoon, again on an empty stomach.

Natural desiccated thyroid may sound ominous, but it is simply thyroid gland tissue from a pig that has been dried and ground into powder. Since the late 1800s when NDT was first created, it has been extremely effective in boosting the body's thyroid levels.

One element that makes NDT so beneficial is that it contains all the thyroid hormones (T1, T2, T3, T4, and calcitonin) that your body needs. Most importantly, the T3-to-T4 ratio of 1 to 4 is the same as it is in your body. Synthetic thyroid medication is only T4 (no active T3 at all) and is a tablet.

Most low-thyroid symptoms, such as fatigue, cold hands, cold feet, brain fog, thinning hair, depressed mood, and weight gain, are usually improved and many times relieved entirely with natural desiccated thyroid or thyroid medications that contain both T4 and T3. However, these symptoms are rarely improved when standard thyroid medication that contains only T4, such as levothyroxine or Synthroid, is prescribed.

I have found most patients get great results with NDT tablets under the tongue (sublingual). This is what June did, and she thrived. These healthy symptoms that describe her today are a long way away from what she used to be. And she loves how she feels today!

Where Hormone Issues Begin

When it comes to hormones, most people probably don't think of the word *thyroid*. Yet it is one of the key hormones—along with the adrenal hormone cortisol and the sex hormone testosterone—and they are all very important at restoring energy to the body. There are several other endocrine (hormone-producing) glands, including the hypothalamus, pancreas, ovaries, testes, pineal gland, pituitary gland, and parathyroid gland.

Remember all the hormone disruptors we talked about earlier? Those disruptors (chemicals, deficiencies, medications, aging, and so on) may affect all your endocrine glands, which in turn negatively impact your hormone levels. The symptoms you develop (such as fatigue or weight gain) usually reflect that impact.

IT'S A FACT

Of the tens of millions of people who suffer from thyroid disease in the USA, 80 percent are women.[1]

The endocrine glands secrete hormones directly into the blood, which is why the application methods (e.g., shots, patches, creams, pellets, sublingual tablets) are important to reach optimal hormone levels in the blood.

Of all the glands, it is the pituitary gland that runs the show. The pituitary secretes thyroid-stimulating hormone (TSH), causing the thyroid gland to make adequate amounts of thyroid hormones. The thyroid knows when sufficient thyroid hormones have been made (to meet the needs of the body and brain), and it relays that information back to the pituitary. This feedback loop is an integral part of your body's health.

These thyroid hormones control the efficiency and speed at which all the cells in your body work.[2] They are incredibly important, sensitive, and complicated, with everything taking place at the cellular level. If there is any miscommunication between the glands and hormones, it is usually reflected in how you feel. That is usually where hormone issues begin.

DEALING WITH SYMPTOMS

Doctors agree on what the thyroid does (regulates heartbeat, manages metabolism, warms you, helps grow hair/nails, restores cells, helps you sleep, and more). They disagree, however, on what to do when symptoms arise.

As you know from experience, most doctors are looking for a way to *patch* (bandage, medicate, comfort) your symptoms. There are unfortunately a lot fewer doctors who look for ways to *fix* (stop, cure, remove) the cause of your symptoms. These are the two main options, and because it is your body, you are the one who gets to choose. If you have hormone symptoms, do you want to *patch* or *fix* them?

For the record, thyroid issues are not new. Back in the 1930s, before World War II, it was estimated that 40 percent of the entire population had thyroid issues![3] And today? As many as 40 percent of Americans are still hypothyroid.[4] I would say that about 50 percent of the US adult population has suboptimal or low normal thyroid levels, but with all the endocrine disruptors today, it may be closer to 60 percent.

You would think that after almost a century of medical advances we would have made some headway! What makes things worse is that we are just talking percentages for those who have thyroid problems. Include the other hormones and the percentage of people with hormone issues only goes higher. Personally, in my thirty-five years of practicing medicine, I would say that most patients who come in with a medical problem also have hormone issues in one way or another. Consider these facts:

- Heart disease is usually a result of hypothyroidism.[5]
- Most women with fertility problems also suffer from hypothyroidism.[6]
- Type 2 diabetics usually suffer from hypothyroidism.[7]
- Alcoholics are usually hypothyroid.[8]
- Chronic infections are usually a sign of hypothyroidism.[9]
- If you suffer from arthritis, you are probably hypothyroid, and your adrenals most likely also need help.[10]
- Hypothyroidism makes every system in the body slow down.[11]
- If you have low T3, then you probably have high cholesterol.[12]
- Cold hands and cold feet are incredibly common, but they are usually a sign the thyroid is sluggish or low. The metabolism isn't functioning well, and weight gain is the natural result.[13]
- Thirty percent of type 1 diabetic women are hypothyroid.[14]

Clearly, patching a symptom does not cure anything. It usually eventually makes things worse, as things compound over time.

Not long ago a patient came in who had Hashimoto's disease (the cause of most hypothyroid cases). She had suffered for years from brain fog, cold hands, cold feet, depression, anxiety, thinning eyebrows, and the inability to lose weight. Her doctor agreed that she had Hashimoto's but said her thyroid numbers were still fine and that he wanted to wait until things got really bad before he started any treatment. In the meantime, medicating the symptoms was the plan, which explained her numerous prescriptions and why her symptoms persisted.

This is not the way to deal with the problem. Until you fix the root cause of the hormone issue, the symptoms will continue, and you will usually get sicker and sicker.

What Are Your Symptoms?

When discussing thyroid problems, we usually hear of *hypothyroidism*, but there is also *hyperthyroidism*. What's the difference? Here's a quick breakdown as well as the most common symptoms of each condition to help you understand.

Hyperthyroidism

This is the overactive thyroid. Think of a cat on catnip! You get random action and plenty of energy but no focus. Interestingly the ratio of females to males of those who suffer from hyperthyroidism is 9 to 1.[15] But overall far fewer people suffer from hyperthyroidism than from hypothyroidism. Symptoms of hyperthyroidism include:

- excessive perspiration
- fatigue
- goiter
- heat intolerance
- hypertension
- menstrual disturbance, light flow
- nervousness, palpitations

- tremor
- weight loss[16]

Hypothyroidism

This is the underactive thyroid. Think of a garden slug moving slowly, not getting much done, but leaving a mess behind. Far more people, both men and women, have hypothyroidism. The symptoms include, but are not limited to:

- acne as an adult
- anxiety and panic attacks
- brain fog
- brittle nails
- carpal tunnel syndrome
- cognitive decline
- cold hands and cold feet
- cold intolerance
- constipation
- cracked heels
- decreased sexual interest
- depression
- downturned mouth
- drooping eyelids
- dry skin, especially on hands, feet, elbows, and knees
- dull facial expression
- ear canal dry, scaly, and itchy
- earwax buildup
- fatigue
- fat pads above clavicles
- fluid retention
- hair loss
- heart disease
- high blood pressure
- high cholesterol
- high cortisol levels
- high insulin levels
- hoarse, husky voice
- inability to concentrate
- infertility
- insomnia
- irritability
- joint pain
- low body temperature
- menstrual irregularities
- migraines
- miscarriage
- muscle and joint pain
- muscle weakness
- puffy face
- ringing in the ears
- swollen eyelids, legs, feet, hands, and belly
- thinning eyebrows
- weight gain[17]

If you have one or two symptoms, then you probably don't have low thyroid. If you have several of these symptoms, you may want to get your thyroid numbers checked, especially your free T3 levels. When patients begin their symptom list with, "I feel bone tired" or "I have no stamina," they invariably nod their heads in agreement to a lot of other symptoms when I mention them. Thankfully all this is fixable, not just patchable.

TESTING YOUR THYROID LEVELS

Before you schedule an appointment for your blood work, I suggest you test yourself at home with the basal body temperature test. Dr. Broda Barnes, one of the top thyroid specialists of all time, used this simple test on his patients with amazing accuracy.

For several days measure your body temperature (thermometer under your arm) every morning before you get out of bed. A normal body temperature hovers around 97.8–98.2°F, so if your average from several mornings is less than 97.8°F, your body is cold. That means your metabolism is running slowly, which is a pretty clear sign of hypothyroidism or suboptimal thyroid function.

When it comes to testing your blood, there are several tests that you should have, including:

- T4
- free T3
- free T4 (optional)
- TSH
- reverse T3 (rT3)

If your body is attacking your thyroid gland (autoimmunity), such as with Hashimoto's, you will have elevated antibodies, so I also recommend testing TPOAbs (thyroid peroxidase) and/or TgAbs (anti-thyroglobulin).

IT'S A FACT

If you have swelling under your skin in the face, jawline, eyelids, and side of your upper arms, test yourself: squeeze the skin on the side of your upper arm. If you pinch skin,

great, but if the skin is thicker or puffy, you may have myx-
edema and have hypothyroidism.

If your doctor won't run these tests for you, find a doctor who will.
(See appendix F.) Why is getting the right test so important? Because
the choice of lab tests and their erroneous normal ranges are the biggest culprit to keeping patients undiagnosed and undertreated![18]

IT'S A FACT

According to the National Institute of Diabetes and Digestive and Kidney Diseases (NIDDK), part of the National
Institutes of Health (NIH), 4.6 percent of the US population age twelve and older has hypothyroidism, although
most cases are mild.[19]

Low- to mid-range thyroid levels are usually going to be associated
with a lot of the symptoms I listed earlier in this chapter, and for those
symptoms you need a remedy, not a patch. That means if you have
symptoms of low thyroid, keep pressing for answers until you get them.

When you mention the need for thyroid testing, almost every doctor
will run the thyroid-stimulating hormone (TSH) test. Some may test
your free T4, but you need all five tests to get an accurate picture of
your thyroid. The TSH test is considered to be the all-knowing gold
standard of thyroid testing by endocrinologists and most doctors, but
there are several details you must know about it.

Fact: TSH measures your pituitary.
The TSH test does indeed measure your thyroid-stimulating hormone, but that is technically a pituitary hormone. It has nothing to do
with what is going on inside your cells, so it cannot accurately reflect
what is happening in your body, but rather what is happening in your
pituitary. The TSH test will indeed show that a small percentage of
people have low thyroid, but for the vast majority, their results will
usually show "normal." An antidepressant or other medication is then
usually recommended.

Doctor Mark Starr went so far as to say, "There is no scientific evidence to support the doctors' claim that the TSH test detects hypothyroidism on the vast majority of patients."[20]

Fact: TSH lacks information.

Sadly the TSH test does not provide you with enough information. You may be experiencing every symptom on the list, but if your numbers are still in range, the TSH test will usually not show you to be hypothyroid. I have no doubt this frustrates millions of people every year.

According to LabCorp, the normal range for adults is 0.45–4.5 µIU/mL (micro–international units per milliliter), but I have found that if your TSH is over 1.0, odds are you have some suboptimal thyroid symptoms. Because of the lack of information, you can feel awful and suffer from countless symptoms but still be diagnosed as having a normal thyroid.

Optimizing thyroid levels will usually reverse the symptoms, but your TSH score may go down to 0.1 µIU/L or lower. That in turn will trigger a red flag with virtually every endocrinologist, and you may be labeled in a "hyperthyroid" state, but that is false. This "below lab range" TSH score is routinely encountered when you are optimally treated with natural thyroid medication.[21]

Optimizing thyroid levels will not make someone hyperthyroid. Most doctors looking at the TSH lab result will believe it does, but that proves the whole point. Optimized T3 levels (with natural desiccated thyroid) will almost always lower the TSH without making you hyperthyroid.

One doctor convinced a patient of mine to stop the optimizing treatment out of fear of atrial fibrillation, a stroke, a heart attack, or osteoporosis. She quit and promptly felt terrible again.

"It will dissolve your bones" or "you will get fractures" or "you will have a heart attack or stroke" are outlived lies, but patients have to choose whether they want to feel great and beat their symptoms or feel mediocre and battle symptoms forever.

Here is the answer: If your TSH numbers go lower than the normal range but you feel good, check your free T3 level. If those numbers are in range, that means you are not hyperthyroid, as many doctors and endocrinologists will assume.

Now, if your free T3 numbers are really high and your pulse is over 100 or you are sweating profusely or have palpitations, then you should lower the dose. Very rarely does this happen. Usually the free T3 numbers are in range and your body feels incredible. Make sure your resting pulse stays less than 100, preferably less than 90.

TOTAL VS. FREE

The thyroid hormones T3 and T4 each have two forms—free and total—and there are different tests to measure each one. In both cases, the test for *free* measures only the thyroid hormone in your body that is available and not bound by proteins, rendering it unable to be used. The test for *total* measures all of that hormone, whether free or protein bound (unusable). Measuring for *free* will give the best picture of your thyroid.

Fact: TSH does not measure the active thyroid hormone.

For a large number of people with thyroid issues, it is a case of their body not producing enough free T3 (the active thyroid hormone that does so much work in your cells). If your TSH score is high (meaning you have low thyroid function), most doctors will prescribe a synthetic thyroid hormone that consists entirely of T4 to normalize (lower) your TSH. I know it's confusing, but if your TSH is high, it means your thyroid function is low.

However, the real issue is not T4; it is free T3 because it is non–protein bound and can easily enter all the cells. Most people with hypothyroid symptoms cannot adequately convert T4 into T3, so dumping more T4 medication into the mix will usually not fix anything. For some more T4 medication will help, but for many people, the symptoms will only persist. The T4 medication will usually normalize the TSH lab value, but it usually does very little in correcting all the low thyroid symptoms.

That is because TSH is a pituitary hormone and not a thyroid hormone. When the thyroid is diseased by Hashimoto's thyroiditis or is low functioning and not producing enough thyroid hormones, TSH levels will usually rise. It's like the pituitary is screaming at the thyroid, "MAKE MORE THYROID HORMONE!"

The thyroid in turn makes more T4 (thyroxine). But the T4 is an inactive hormone and needs to be converted to T3 (the active thyroid hormone). T3 must be unbound from its protein to become free T3 so that it can enter all the cells.

Most doctors rely on the TSH test (remember, the normal range for LabCorp is 0.45–4.5 µIU/mL), and if the TSH is over 4.5, the patient is low thyroid, and if the TSH is less than 0.45, the patient is hyperthyroid. Sadly there are millions of patients with low and suboptimal thyroid who are not treated as a result.

Again, a much more accurate test is measuring the free T3 level, and then I recommend optimizing that level to 3.5–4.4 pg/mL and sometimes slightly higher. Free T3 is the active form of thyroid that resolves most symptoms of low thyroid when it is optimized. You could have a normal T4 (the inactive thyroid hormone) and very low free T3 and still have a "normal" TSH level. The TSH test misses many patients with low, sluggish, and suboptimal thyroid function.

As you can see, it's impossible for the TSH test to give a full diagnosis of your thyroid issues. So what does the TSH test tell you? It tests your pituitary hormone as part of the thyroid-pituitary-hypothalamic loop, so you will know if your pituitary gland is functioning well or not. Finding that out is helpful, but it is not going to address your other thyroid issues at all.

SYNTHETIC THYROID TO THE RESCUE

To combat the ever-growing thyroid problem stemming from iodine deficiency, which affects about 40 percent of the total earth's population,[22] a pharmaceutical company in the 1950s created Synthroid. It became, and still is, one of the most prescribed medications in the United States. In 2016 it was the most prescribed drug, with 123 million prescriptions that year.[23]

When Synthroid made its debut, natural desiccated thyroid was widely used. The owners of Synthroid paid a researcher to show how Synthroid was superior to natural desiccated thyroid. The researcher found the opposite to be true, but the company blocked her story and tried to discredit her. Eventually the truth came out: natural desiccated thyroid (NDT) is more effective than Synthroid.[24]

One of the primary reasons NDT outperforms synthetic Synthroid is that NDT matches your body's 1-to-4 ratio of T3 to T4. Synthroid's only ingredient is non-active T4.

IT'S A FACT

I believe the obesity epidemic follows the thyroid epidemic. Some argue the obesity epidemic is bringing with it a new wave of hormone problems, and that is true as well.

To conceptualize what is happening here with T4 and T3 at the cellular level, imagine a grandfather who has a knack for building birdhouses. They are cute and colorful and come in a range of sizes. But let's say he builds them and puts them in his garage. Once that is full, he fills the attic, then the bedrooms, and eventually there is no more room for another birdhouse.

What he should be doing is taking the birdhouses outside and putting them to use so they can be filled with birds. The active element, the very thing that makes a birdhouse a birdhouse, is missing when all you do is jam the house full of birdhouses. Fill them with birds, and suddenly you have action, purpose, and life.

That is T4 to T3. The T4 is a storehouse—a mini storage unit, if you will—but filling your body with T4 will not usually fix you. Odds are, you need adequate active T3. In fact, your body requires a ratio of 1 to 4 (T3 to T4). Yes, T4 can help with some patients who are able to convert T4 to T3. However, most patients cannot adequately or optimally convert T4 to T3 because of nutritional deficiencies, chronic stress, medications, diseases, diet, fluoride, age, hormone disruptors, chlorine, and so on.

Synthroid then went on the offensive and perpetuated a hoax that the desiccated thyroid was unreliably mixed, scaring patients with the fear that the dosage might be too little or too much. Eventually it was shown that Synthroid was the one unreliably mixed (the FDA has pulled the product from the shelves several times for this very reason),[25] but by the time the facts were known, doctors en masse had already pulled their patients off natural desiccated thyroid and put them on Synthroid.

Guess what happened to the patients who had been controlling their symptoms with NDT? Exactly! It's likely that all of their negative symptoms returned. Metaphorically speaking, tens of thousands of birdhouses were shaken clean and returned to attics across the nation. Thousands of people lived with fatigue, cold hands and cold feet, brain fog, continued weight gain, and many of the other symptoms of hypo-thyroidism. The joy and sounds of life were silenced. And the dreary, depressed life returned.

You would think the fact that patients' symptoms returned as soon as they replaced the natural thyroid with a synthetic would have been enough to sway public opinion in favor of what actually works. You would think that, but doctors, endocrinologists, and pharmaceutical companies maintained that synthetic was the only way to go. That is still the standard preference, but you will find more and more doctors who are using natural desiccated thyroid to treat hypothyroid patients.

SYNTHETIC ANSWERS ARE NOT WORKING

After decades of synthetic T4 thyroid medication, patients are told their persistent symptoms are normal, as if there is nothing you can do to fix them. The T4-only approach to treating thyroid issues leaves quite a few symptoms behind. This list is incredible.

Symptoms while on T4-only medications:

- aching bones/muscles/joints
- cold backside
- cold hands and cold feet
- constipation
- cracked heels
- depression
- dry hair and skin
- exhaustion
- forgetfulness/fogginess
- hair loss and breakage
- hard, little, round stools
- heavy-feeling arms after activity
- heavy periods
- high cholesterol
- inability to concentrate
- inability to get pregnant
- irritability
- lack of energy
- lack of sex drive
- lack of stamina
- loss of appetite
- need for naps
- ridged fingernails
- ringing in the ears
- thinning eyebrows
- thin skin
- weight gain[26]

Yes, you guessed it; not much has changed! What your body needs is adequate amounts of active T3. That will usually take care of most hypothyroid issues, including everything on this T4-only symptom list.

One primary reason why the T4-only approach does not work well is because excessive T4 usually causes your body to make reverse T3 (rT3) from the active T3 hormones in an effort to get rid of the extra T4.[27] What this means is that your body dumps the excess T4 by wasting your good and active T3. Using the birdhouse analogy, rT3 locks the birdhouse closed. All you can do is throw it away at that point. The only good thing about rT3 is you are clearing out the house so you have room for more, but the bad news is that the birdhouses you throw out can never be used properly.

Excessive T4 usually eventually means extra rT3, but your body requires approximately a 20-to-1 ratio of free T3 to rT3 or higher. When you get below that ratio, you usually start to develop symptoms on the T4-only list. Keep up the imbalance of free T3 to rT3 (less than a 20-to-1 ratio) and chronic illnesses usually set in. We are talking about fibromyalgia, chronic fatigue, obesity, type 2 diabetes, chronic pain syndromes, and more. Chronic conditions usually only make the imbalance all the more severe over time.

High rT3 is nothing to mess with, yet the TSH test will give you a "normal range" lab result! That is why you need to test for rT3 as well as free T3. Knowing both, you can then calculate your ratio. To calculate your free T3-to-rT3 ratio, use an online calculator such as https://stopthethyroidmadness.com/rt3-ratio. Make sure you select the correct units of measurement for both free T3 and rT3.

THE HORMONE HEALTH ZONE FOR THYROID HEALTH

The hormone health zone for your thyroid is pretty well-defined. The goals are:

- Maximize T4-to-T3 conversion.
- Lower rT3 to maintain a 20-to-1 ratio of free T3 to rT3 or higher.

When that is the case, all the symptoms of hypothyroidism usually stop, rewind, and fade away. When you optimize your thyroid levels, all these pieces come together. You have sufficient T4-to-T3 conversion, the ratio of T3 to rT3 is 20 to 1 or higher, and you have plenty of active T3 at work in your body.

If you have thyroid symptoms, but they are not going away, you have not yet optimized your thyroid at one level or another. It's as simple as that.

For me, my sluggish thyroid meant brain fog, cold hands, cold feet, decreased energy, and afternoon naps. My TSH was normal at 1.0 µIU/mL even though I felt horrible with many of the symptoms listed above. But my symptoms were all cleared up when I raised my free T3 from 2.5 pg/mL to 4.0 pg/mL. The normal range is 2.0–4.4 pg/mL, and I was in the normal range all along, but the symptoms did not go away until I optimized my T3 levels specifically.

Maximizing T4 to T3 for more active T3

I put my patients who need to increase their free T3 levels (by maximizing the T4-to-T3 conversion process) on natural desiccated thyroid and recheck their free T3 in two to four weeks. If their level is better, they usually feel better, feel warmer, look brighter, and are happier. We turn it up a bit, but not too fast. "Start low and go slow" is the best method.

I have patients check their pulse daily as well as their auxiliary temperature morning and evening. If their pulse goes over 100, I will usually lower their dose of thyroid and continue monitoring their free T3.

Patients over sixty-five and anyone who has heart disease needs to start very low and go very slow on thyroid, or small to moderate doses of thyroid could stress their heart. One ninety-year-old patient had a free T3 of 1.2 and a normal TSH. I slowly raised her thyroid dose, and her free T3 was 2.2. When I tried to raise it further, her pulse went to 120, so I had to back it down, and she's doing great.

A few weeks or months later, if there's not much change in symptoms, we then check the rT3. The rT3 may be blocking the T4-to-T3 conversion.

The overall process of raising active free T3 is pretty simple, yet highly effective. Free T3 is active and plays such a vital role in your health, so when the numbers go up, you usually feel it! For more information, see appendix D, "How to Maximize Your T4-to-T3 Conversion."

Lowering rT3

To lower your body's rT3, you need to only take liothyronine thyroid in the form of T3. You don't need any more T4, as you already have T4 in excess. Taking T3 only automatically starts lowering your T4 levels, which lowers rT3 as well. (Find a physician who is knowledgeable in this area from appendix F.)

I recommend starting with 5 mcg (micrograms) of T3 (liothyronine) twice a day (if you are sensitive, you may need to start with 2.5 mcg) and increasing the dosage every three to four days slowly until you are at 25 mcg twice a day; then stay at that dose for about three months. Monitor your pulse two to three times each day along the way. Make sure your pulse does not go over 100 while resting or that you have no palpitations or irregular heartbeats. If you do, decrease your dose, and that usually corrects the problem. Remain under the care of a physician who knows how to lower rT3 by using this method.

Take a multivitamin as well as the supplement selenium (100–200 mg once per day). Eating according to the Keto Zone diet (see appendix F) or an anti-inflammatory, gluten-free diet is recommended. For more information, see appendix E, "How to Lower Your rT3 Levels," and appendix F to find a physician.

Your Optimized Thyroid Levels

The recommended tests and the normal ranges are as follows:

> free T3: 2.0–4.4 pg/mL
>
> free T4: 0.8–1.8 ng/dL (optional)
>
> TSH: 0.45–4.5 μIU/L
>
> rT3: less than 15 ng/dL
>
> antibodies—TPOAbs or TgAbs: 10–20 IU/ml

When your thyroid levels are optimized, your numbers will be closer to these:

free T3: 3.5–4.4 pg/mL

free T4: 1.2–1.8 ng/dL (optional)

TSH: 0.1–1.0 μIU/L or lower

rT3: less than 15 ng/dL (based on the 20-to-1 ratio)

antibodies—TPOAbs or TgAbs: less than 10 IU/mL

free T3-to-rT3 ratio: 20 to 1 or higher

I believe the most important numbers to know, track, and manage with your thyroid are your free T3, rT3, and TPO levels. Therefore, testing for free T3 and rT3 is critical. Most doctors do not even test for those numbers, so be sure that you request them.

Hypothyroidism or suboptimal thyroid levels affect many of us, which means you can probably identify with several of the symptoms listed earlier in this chapter. Thankfully you can fix this! The symptoms do not need to define you or your life.

CHAPTER 9

ADRENAL RESTORATION

I N MY BOOK *Stress Less* I share a story about a house on a lake my family owned years ago. After we sold it, my son and nephew (both teenagers at the time) accompanied my wife on a quick trip to retrieve a small paddleboat we had left behind at a neighbor's house on the lake.

It was to be a simple errand, but when they arrived, a neighbor's pit bull on the second-story balcony started barking wildly. The closer they came, the more berserk it went. Finally the dog jumped over the railing to the ground below and raced toward them in a full-on rage.

My son took off running down the dock and jumped in the lake. The dog followed him in and dog-paddled after him. Thinking quickly, my son took off a shoe and hit the dog several times on the head. Eventually the dog got frustrated and swam back to shore.

My nephew, big and strong and hoping to get into the Marines, was standing on the shore. As soon as that pit bull came out of the water, it went after my nephew. Taking a defensive posture, my nephew went into attack mode as well. When the dog lunged at him, he would hit it in the head with his fist. The dog would just shake his head and attack again and again. Eventually, however, the dog was able to bite his thigh.

At this point Mary started yelling, "Don't look at him in the eyes! Don't look at him in the eyes!" She had seen a special on TV a few weeks earlier that had explained how if you are ever attacked by a dog, you should not look at the dog in the eyes. It usually infuriates them. Instead, tuck in your extremities, turn your back, and avoid eye contact. At least that was what the commentator had said.

The dog let go of my nephew's leg and charged across the lawn toward my wife, who was about fifty yards away on a little hill. What should she do? Run? Jump in the lake? Hit the dog? Hoping and praying the documentary was true, she folded her arms in and turned her back to the dog. As the dog ran around her, barking and growling and trying to get eye contact, she would turn like a top to avoid eye contact.

In what seemed like hours but was only minutes, the police and several neighbors arrived, and the dog was contained. Afterward, Mary brought everyone straight to my office. My nephew had a few superficial lacerations on his thigh, which I cleaned and bandaged.

I noticed the boys joking with each other, laughing and talking about how crazy it was and what they both did to escape. They were using words like *cool* and *neat* to describe their harrowing experience. I checked, and their blood pressure and heart rates were also normal.

Mary, on the other hand, was not using similar words to describe the ordeal! She sat in the office chair, visibly shaking. Her arms were folded around her chest in the same position as when she was avoiding eye contact with the pit bull, her fists were clenched, and her blood pressure and heart rate were elevated.

"Try to relax," I directed.

"I can't," she replied.

"Everything turned out fine," I encouraged.

"I know," she acknowledged, "but I keep seeing that dog charging after me, and I still hear his growling."

That made me consider their responses. When we are faced with sudden danger, our natural response is fight or flight. Our bodies produce a surge of adrenaline, and we take action.

- My son fled. That was his response, and that action burned off the adrenaline, the main stress hormone. His body was able to reset its stress-response mechanism. He was fine. His body reflected that.

- My nephew fought back. That response also burned off the excess adrenaline. His stress-response mechanism also reset.

- But Mary did not fight or flee. Instead, she stood there. Now, running or fighting would probably have resulted in her getting attacked by that dog, so for her own safety her choice of following the documentary's direction of avoiding eye contact did indeed protect her.

However, when that pit bull turned its attention on her and starting charging, her body had a surge of adrenaline. Because she neither fought nor fled, adrenaline was pumping through her body and caused her stress response to become stuck in sympathetic dominance, similar to an accelerator on a car that is stuck to the floor. She was still "stewing" in the mix of adrenaline and cortisol several hours after the attack. Her stress-response mechanism could not reset because it had never been shut off and she was reliving the attack.

What made this experience even more interesting was that we were scheduled to go on a cruise the following week. For the first few days on the cruise I would find her in a chair with her fists clenched and arms pulled up.

"Mary, you need to relax," I would say.

"Oh, I didn't realize I was doing that," she would reply.

This happened repeatedly.

During our week onboard the ship, we went to comedy clubs, talked with friends, and enjoyed our time together. Finally she began to unwind, especially after having a hot stone massage.

We also talked it through. She reframed the situation. Instead of thinking, "I almost got killed by a pit bull!" she reframed it to, "Thank you, God, for keeping me safe, keeping everyone safe, and for showing me that TV show just weeks before the attack."

Relaxing plus reframing the situation helped her reset her stress-response mechanism. It took her almost a week to reach the same state that my nephew and son had attained in less than an hour after their attacks. If she had not reframed the situation and reset her stress response, she probably would have developed post traumatic stress disorder, or PTSD. I felt it was worth sharing that story again in this chapter because it perfectly illustrates the important role stress plays in all of our daily lives.

Following the Adrenaline Trail

Not everyone has heard about the adrenal glands, but everyone has heard about adrenaline. This famous fight-or-flight hormone (also called epinephrine) gives your body and muscles a boost (extra blood flow, heart pumping, eye dilation, and blood sugar released) when you really need it. Blood is diverted away from the skin and digestive tract and shunted to the muscles and brain.

The adrenal glands (there are two of them, right above your kidneys) not only produce adrenaline; they also produce cortisol, among several other hormones. It is cortisol that plays a big role in your endocrine system.

At first glance it would seem pretty simple to diagnose adrenal gland issues. Too much cortisol being produced can lead to Cushing's syndrome, and not enough cortisol production can lead to Addison's disease.

- Cushing's syndrome: Symptoms include truncal obesity; round, red face; high blood pressure; acne; sarcopenia; osteoporosis; thin skin; PMS; mood swings; chronic fatigue; migraines; and more. The cause of Cushing's syndrome: usually a tumor in the adrenal glands or cortisone-like medications.

IT'S A FACT

JFK suffered from Addison's disease.

- Addison's disease: Symptoms advance slowly over time and include weight loss, muscle weakness, muscle/joint pain, dark spots on your skin (or even your gums), low blood pressure, nausea, low libido, fainting, and more. The cause of Addison's disease: tuberculosis, infections of the adrenal glands, spread of cancer to the adrenal glands, or most commonly autoimmune disease.

Cortisol is produced to help the body respond to stress. Small increases in cortisol will usually give you a burst of energy, improve memory and immunity, and even lower your sensitivity to pain. The stress response may have produced adrenaline to get you going, but your body needs cortisol to help respond to stress in a healthy manner. Nobody should stay in a heightened state (heard of the term *adrenaline junky*?) because it's not healthy.

Only a very small number of people suffer from Cushing's or Addison's, so you probably don't need to worry about either of those conditions. Both illnesses are treatable by optimizing hormone levels and correcting the underlying problem, should you need to address either of them. If it isn't Cushing's or Addison's that concerns the vast majority of the US population, what makes the adrenals—and the cortisol hormone in particular—so important? The adrenals are vital because the ongoing long-term effect of the adrenal glands pumping out excessive cortisol repeatedly during the day for minor stresses may eventually damage and destroy our bodies.

Several years ago researchers wrote that a mild degree of cortisol overproduction by the adrenals, without any noticeable symptoms, was more common than Cushing's or Addison's.[1] They were right about Cushing's and Addison's being not very common, but they were very wrong about mild overproduction leaving no obvious symptoms behind. That is the adrenaline trail, and it is leading millions of people off a health-ruining cliff!

THE ROLE OF ADRENALS IN YOUR HEALTH

When it comes to your adrenals, hormones, and overall health, I have come to this conclusion: you will never balance—much less optimize—your other hormones until you balance your adrenal hormones. Quite simply, your hormone health requires healthy adrenals. That is because impaired adrenal function can make your hormone issues worse and delay any forward progress you might be making. Sometimes the adrenals are the root of the problem, but usually they act more like gas or accelerant to an already-burning fire. They usually make things worse, and putting a fire out with gas is not a good strategy.

IT'S A FACT

Adrenal fatigue has similar symptoms to Addison's disease but usually in a milder manner.

Most doctors don't even test the adrenals, which can explain why so many adrenal issues are missed. When the plan is to address an issue only when it's bad enough, then an adrenal test is of little value. When the plan is to fix/prevent rather than patch/cover, getting your adrenals checked just might shed some light on your symptoms and possible hormone issues.

As I have briefly discussed, the adrenals give you adrenaline and cortisol to help your body respond to stress. But long-term exposure to cortisol negatively impacts your body, and it's connected to what I discussed in the previous chapter about thyroid hormones and will discuss in future chapters on other hormones. Allow me to explain.

1. Excessive cortisol blocks T4-to-T3 conversion. Yes, you read that correctly. The vital conversion process that gives your body its much-needed active T3 thyroid hormone is slowed down sometimes significantly by the extra cortisol in your system. You could literally be hypothyroid, with the many unpleasant symptoms that go with it, all because your adrenals are producing too much cortisol.

2. Excessive cortisol increases rT3 production. Increasing the production of rT3 in your body wrecks the necessary 20-to-1 ratio of free T3 to rT3, and that in turn usually results in a very sick thyroid. Some nasty hypothyroid symptoms and chronic diseases are right behind it. Of course that in turn only makes things worse.

3. Excessive cortisol lowers testosterone. This also is big news! In the following chapters I will discuss the importance of testosterone for both men and women, but for now, suffice it to say that you absolutely do not want to lower testosterone levels. The symptoms of low testosterone are some of the worst.

4. Excessive cortisol increases conversion of testosterone into estrogen. Men certainly don't want more estrogen in their bodies, but neither do women want this type of estrogen elevated. The

type of estrogen created is usually estrone, which is the so-called "old lady estrogen" that usually causes more belly fat and weight gain. The testosterone-to-estrogen balance is vital for both men and women, but cortisol ruins it. I will discuss more about estrogen for men and women in later chapters.

Because most hormones operate in a feedback loop, the lower your hormones go, usually the more cortisol you make, and the more cortisol your body pumps out, the more it messes up your other hormones.

This vicious cycle never ends, but your adrenals cannot keep it up forever. The overproduction of cortisol eventually wears your adrenal glands down, resulting in adrenal fatigue and even complete adrenal burnout. Cortisol levels usually plummet, which increases your risk for inflammatory and autoimmune diseases and essentially invites them into your body.

The negative impact of blocked T4-to-T3 conversion, increased rT3 production, lowered testosterone, and testosterone turning into estrogen makes for a hodgepodge list of symptoms nobody wants to identify with. Unfortunately doctors see these symptoms walk in the door every day and frequently diagnose them as obesity, dementia, osteoporosis, sarcopenia, hypertension, depression, fibromyalgia, or type 2 diabetes, but completely miss the root cause, which is adrenal burnout, or adrenal fatigue. The symptoms include:

- weight gain
- brain fog
- depression
- memory issues
- constant fatigue

But wait, there is more—as if this wasn't enough! When your adrenals are tired, they produce less of the antiaging hormone dihydroepiandosterone (DHEA). This is another hormone made in your adrenal glands whose role it is to help your body build muscle and keep you looking and feeling young.

The problem for all of us is that after age twenty our DHEA levels drop by about 2 percent each year.[2] But if you speed up the DHEA decline by adding adrenal fatigue, you naturally get lower DHEA hormone levels sooner than normal. These low levels come with their own list of symptoms:

- chronic infections
- heart disease
- insomnia
- cancers
- arthritis
- Alzheimer's
- Parkinson's
- lupus
- accelerated aging
- wrinkles and sagging skin

As you can see, your adrenals play a pivotal role in your overall health. If your adrenal glands are hurting, so are you.

What Causes Adrenal Fatigue?

You may be thinking, "I'm not an adrenaline junky, and I don't have daily scary situations that get my adrenaline pumping, so why would my adrenals even have an issue?"

I admit, scary adrenaline-pumping moments are few and far between, and thankfully so. However, your body is under other pressures, stressors, and worries that never give your stress-response system a break. Cortisol is naturally produced to calm things down in short-term, high-alert situations. When there is no end to the loop or the stress, the cortisol keeps flowing. It's like your alarm button is stuck in the "on" position, and cortisol levels get higher and higher.

High cortisol can disrupt important bodily functions and lead to problems such as high blood sugar, high blood pressure, decreased thyroid function, and adrenal fatigue. (See the symptoms of adrenal fatigue listed elsewhere in this chapter.)

All of us experience stress. There's no way to avoid it entirely. So what do we do? I have found that most people dealing with adrenal issues from stress fall into one of the following categories:

Type 1: Super-busy people—These are often type A people who are go-getters. They work hard, have crazy hours, juggle everything, are super busy, and live with far too many things on their plates.

Type 2: Good people dealing with bad situations—The average person is under constant daily stress from finances, the job, marriage, children, traffic, and relationships. The stress burden becomes unbearable when you add any other high-stress major life events such as the death of a loved one, a divorce, marital separation, a break-up, a move, a serious illness, an accident, domestic abuse, or a job loss.

Type 3: Sick people—These are people with chronic illness (e.g., fibromyalgia), chronic pain, inflammation, panic attacks, anxiety, depression, chronic fatigue, chronic Lyme disease, mold illness, insomnia, or PTSD. They are burned out, frazzled, sick, and hurting, and they can't sleep.

Which are you? Do any of these descriptions fit you, your personality, or your situation? You and your doctor will need to confirm this, but from the many patients who have come through my door over the past thirty-five years, I would say that if you are type 1 or type 2, you most likely have adrenal fatigue. If you are type 3 and battle anything chronic, then your adrenals are most likely burned out and maybe even flatlined.

Generally speaking, we all fit into one of these three types, and that means we are all tiring our adrenals out. We need to recharge and reboot our adrenals, or we will have a host of symptoms and diseases to deal with later down the road. I have even seen teenagers suffering from adrenal burnout. That is no way to head into the future. And that is why my experience practicing medicine tells me this cortisol loop applies to us all.

Enough has probably been said about the adrenals for you to accurately tell if you have adrenal fatigue. But here is a ranking test that may help you clarify for yourself even more. Go ahead and rate yourself.

ADRENAL FATIGUE			
SYMPTOM	RATE IT		
	0 (NEVER)	1 (OCCASIONALLY)	2 (OFTEN)	3 (ALWAYS)
Anxiety and panic attacks	0	1	2	3
Anxiety or nervousness	0	1	2	3
Blood pressure increases	0	1	2	3
Brain fog	0	1	2	3
Cold hands and cold feet	0	1	2	3
Constant fatigue	0	1	2	3
Decline in enjoyment in life	0	1	2	3
Decreased work performance	0	1	2	3
Depression	0	1	2	3
Dizziness or light-headedness (especially when going from a seated or lying position to standing)	0	1	2	3
Dry, thin skin that doesn't heal quickly	0	1	2	3
Fluid retention	0	1	2	3
Flushed face or sweat	0	1	2	3
Grumpiness	0	1	2	3
Hair loss, including eyebrows	0	1	2	3
Headaches	0	1	2	3
Heart disease	0	1	2	3
Inability to focus	0	1	2	3
Inability to handle life	0	1	2	3
Inability to sleep	0	1	2	3
Infertility and miscarriage	0	1	2	3
Insomnia	0	1	2	3
Irritability	0	1	2	3
Lowered sex drive	0	1	2	3
Memory issues	0	1	2	3
Menstrual irregularities	0	1	2	3

ADRENAL FATIGUE				
SYMPTOM	**RATE IT**			
	0 (NEVER)	1 (OCCASIONALLY)	2 (OFTEN)	3 (ALWAYS)
Muscle and joint pain	0	1	2	3
Muscle weakness	0	1	2	3
Need for frequent naps	0	1	2	3
Prediabetic and diabetic symptoms	0	1	2	3
Rapid heart rate	0	1	2	3
Rising cholesterol	0	1	2	3
Road rage	0	1	2	3
Sensitive eyes	0	1	2	3
Sweets or salt craving	0	1	2	3
Tiredness upon waking up	0	1	2	3
Weight gain	0	1	2	3

If you scored over forty, you should consider doing a salivary adrenal test. (See adrenal testing in appendix F and later in this chapter.) These symptoms of adrenal fatigue, along with other symptoms of sluggish thyroid and suboptimal testosterone levels, combine to form a toxic mix of pains and ailments that are typically treated with antidepressants, antianxiety meds, insomnia meds, and other medications. Only when you address the true cause are you able to break free and help your adrenals get the rest they need and recharge.

TEST YOUR ADRENAL HEALTH

There are several ways to screen your adrenals, and you may want to do more than one test to confirm the results. I have found the following three tests to be very accurate, noninvasive, and easy to do.

Adrenal test 1: seven-day temperature test

You can do this test at home, and it is also a good way to check your thyroid. Take your temperature every three hours, starting when you wake up. If you are eating or exercising at the three-hour mark, wait thirty minutes before checking your temperature. You are looking for any variation between your numbers.

If your daily body temperature average is 98.6°F, which is normal, but if you fluctuated 0.2–0.3° between measurements, then your adrenals probably have an issue but not your thyroid. However, if your temperature is below normal, but steady, then it's more likely a thyroid issue, and your adrenals may be fine. All combined (low temperature with fluctuations) means you most likely have both adrenal and thyroid issues.

Adrenal test 2: saliva test

Cortisol levels fluctuate during the day, so the saliva test collects your saliva four to six times in a day, then gives you an average cortisol score. Basically you spit in a plastic vial every four hours. Like the seven-day temperature test, wait thirty minutes after food or exercise. Then send the vial by mail to the medical service provider. I believe this is more accurate than a blood test for two reasons: (1) a blood test only measures your cortisol levels once, and they could simply be high or low at that moment, and (2) the needle prick from a blood test causes enough stress to affect cortisol levels, but there is no stress in a saliva test. (See appendix F for more information about the saliva test.)

Adrenal test 3: blood pressure screening test

The blood pressure test is usually done in a doctor's office. While lying down, check your blood pressure. Then check it while you are standing. Normally your blood pressure should increase 10–20 points when standing. If your blood pressure drops by 10 points or more, you probably have low adrenal function. Usually the greater the drop, the lower the adrenal function.

Because there are many recommended tests for adrenals, you will have to choose the one you prefer. I usually recommend the blood pressure screen and the saliva test because it only takes one day to complete both of these. At the mention of adrenal testing, most doctors will recommend the adrenocorticotropic hormone (ACTH) stimulation test or more tests, such as a blood serum/cortisol test or a twenty-four-hour urine collection test for cortisol. Unfortunately none of these three tests give the best results for showing adrenal fatigue.

SLEEP APNEA AND ADRENALS

It is not just a nuisance. If you suffer from sleep apnea, your brain is likely starved for oxygen, and you have unknowingly signed up for almost every disease. Take a moment to answer:

- Do you snore at night? Y/N
- Do you stop breathing at night? Y/N
- Do you wake up gasping for air? Y/N
- Do you have a dry mouth in the morning? Y/N

People with sleep apnea are usually bone tired, have no energy, and cannot seem to get recharged. That is adrenal fatigue in action. They also have a higher risk for high blood pressure, memory loss, atrial fibrillation, diabetes, cancer, heart issues, dementia, and more, all because of the lack of oxygen. If you have sleep apnea, you cannot make it into the hormone health zone. You are stuck. You must break free of sleep apnea first.

- **Step 1** is to get more oxygen with a CPAP (or BiPAP) machine. Armed with sufficient oxygen, the adrenals do not have to work as hard, blood pressure comes down, and losing weight is easier.
- **Step 2** is to use diet (e.g., the Keto Zone diet) and moderate exercise to assist the healing process.
- **Step 3** is to optimize hormone levels. Many patients eventually do away with their CPAP machines entirely at that point.

THE MIND-SET OF ADRENAL HEALTH

When you exercise a muscle, and it is sore the next day, you rest it for a few days, and that is usually sufficient. Very simple. The same process of resting is needed for your adrenal glands, but that cannot happen if you are in the never-ending loop of cortisol production.

The answer is to address the root issues that cause adrenal fatigue. Then your body can shake off the symptoms. For me, I was the super-busy, type A person. I worked crazy long hours, tried to meet the needs of forty to fifty patients every day, managed a growing practice, wrote books, spoke in churches and on TV and the radio in my "off" time, and exercised every weekday. Basically I burned the candle at both ends.

I was far too busy. All combined to tire out my adrenals, which, technically speaking, hurt my T4-to-T3 conversion and lowered my active T3, and I developed symptoms accordingly. How did I fix the real problem? I had to learn how to:

- say no more than I said yes
- not get in a hurry
- slow down
- get into God's rhythm and stay there (It's a flow.)
- breathe, relax, and go with the flow
- not push and strive
- not fight the riptide of life

I also stopped working on Saturdays, stopped taking calls in the middle of the night, and saw fewer patients. My psoriasis, IBS, chronic fatigue, and chronic sinusitis were stressing my adrenals as well. I actually needed small doses of cortisol to help reboot my system. Because my adrenals and cortisol levels were almost flatlined, pushing my adrenals way too far and dealing with chronic illness, it took me six to nine months to reboot my adrenal glands.

Overall, dealing with adrenal glands includes the element of mental changes, behavioral therapy, and reframing work, and that holds true for all of us. Most of our stresses are mental and emotional stress. Seldom is it only physical.

Twelve Secrets to a Healthy Adrenal Mind-Set

Patients with adrenal issues will find relief and healing when they have a mind-set that promotes adrenal health. Here are twelve secrets to a healthy adrenal mind-set.

1. **Reframe stresses.** Like Mary with the dog attack, reframing the incident helped her considerably.

2. **Forgive.** A single moment of unforgiveness, whatever the cause, can hold people captive.

3. **Deal honestly with issues.** Even half-stresses are perceived stresses.

4. **Apply eye movement desensitization and reprocessing (EMDR).** Specialists in EMDR can help heal the impact of traumas that keep your stress response stuck and cause anxiety, panic attacks, and PTSD.

5. **Learn to manage and budget.** When problems are managed, be they financial, relational, or other, they are not as bad. Especially manage your finances, and avoid going into debt.

6. **Get counseling.** A listening ear, with good practical advice, is a great help.

7. **Change thinking through cognitive behavioral therapy.** A professional counselor can help you correct flawed thinking that brings pain and stress. For example, when someone believes others are against him, everything will be seen through that light.

8. **Let go.** Anger, resentment, and disappointment need to be released for good.

9. **Laugh at life.** Life happens, so you might as well laugh along the way. I commonly prescribe ten belly laughs a day!

10. **Live in peace.** Keep your heart, mind, and body at peace, and spend at least fifteen minutes first thing in the morning reading your Bible.

11. **Give yourself room.** Practice having extra margins or breathing room in all areas of your life. Give yourself enough time and space to get things done.

12. **Filter thoughts and actions through God's Word.** Philippians 4:8 commands us to think on things that are true, noble, just, pure, lovely, and of good report. Refuse to think on anything contrary to that, and run every thought through that filter. If the thought is not pure, then don't think on it, and let it go.

You have probably seen the famous Serenity Prayer by American theologian Reinhold Niebuhr. When I was younger, I thought it was something older people might say. The truth is, it's 100 percent applicable to all of us:

> God, grant me the serenity to accept the things I cannot change, courage to change the things I can, and wisdom to know the difference.

The enemy of your adrenals is excessive, unrelenting stress, which comes in countless forms. Your job is to find what gives you the upper hand and then learn to live that way.

TREATMENT PLAN FOR ADRENAL HEALTH

Another important detail few know is that our stress-response system is basically like a timer. After the adrenaline boost, it takes about ninety minutes for it to reset. If you reset it (e.g., fight or flight, address the issue, choose to forgive, reframe it, move on, walk in peace, and so on), then the timer turns off. If you don't stop it, the timer will keep on ticking, and cortisol levels may stay elevated. This can go on for years until your adrenals crash and you develop adrenal fatigue with low cortisol levels.

Whenever you choose to remain too busy, multitasking, moving too fast, offended, angry, depressed, and so on, you allow the timer to keep running. You must learn how to stop the timer and then learn how to treat your adrenals. In addition to the mental and emotional side of adrenal health, there is the practical treatment side as well, which includes:

Sleep and rest

- Get a good night's sleep: seven to nine hours and some-times ten hours each night for those with severe adrenal fatigue.
- Learn to rest. Find things you enjoy doing that make you feel recharged.
- Overcome insomnia with natural supplements such as melatonin, L-theanine, magnesium threonate, or micronized progesterone for women.

Diet

- The Keto Zone diet or Let Food Be Your Medicine diet (see appendix F) or a similar anti-inflammatory diet is ideal.
- Drink a lot of alkaline water (at least one to two quarts).
- Avoid excessive caffeine.

Nutrition

- Include vitamin supplements (B_5, C, and D), sele-nium, iodine, iron for women, zinc, magnesium, and B complex.
- Adaptogens or adaptogenic herbs can balance (increase or decrease) cortisol levels, based on your body's needs, and that is healthy. Some natural adaptogenic herbs include ginseng (American, Asian, or Siberian), rho-diola, ashwagandha, licorice, rhaponticum, reishi, and many more.
- Adrenal glandular extracts from pig, sheep, or cow are adrenal rebuilders in pill form and may be taken one

to three times a day. You can usually get them in most
health food stores.

- Myers' IV (contains vitamins and minerals that help support and reboot the adrenals; usually given once a week)

Exercise

Find an exercise program you enjoy, one that does not burn all the little energy you have left. If you are suffering from severe adrenal fatigue, very mild exercises are recommended, such as stretching and leisurely walks as able (not necessarily daily) for only ten to thirty minutes. If exercise leaves you exhausted, decrease your time and intensity of exercise. You should feel refreshed after exercising and not exhausted. Some patients with severe adrenal fatigue need to wait a few months before exercising to help recharge their adrenals.

SIDE EFFECTS

There are no negative side effects from decreasing the effects of stress in your life. It really is controlling how you react to stress that is the main issue behind adrenal health.

Some patients have adrenal issues and no thyroid problems at all. All they usually need is a good multivitamin with adequate B vitamins, especially B_5, and maybe some rhodiola (an adaptogen) and to follow the above treatment plan for adrenal health.

For most people who suffer from adrenal fatigue, the combination of mental adrenal health with these practical elements will be enough to recharge their adrenals. Yes, it will typically take a few months to a year to get their adrenals back to normal, but it's a process as well as new habit formation.

But when people have pushed their adrenal fatigue to the level of adrenal exhaustion, they will usually need additional help to reboot their adrenal glands. This also happens to people who are chronically ill (with fibromyalgia, Lyme disease, cancer, and so on). The severity of their illness is what drains their adrenals.

Whatever the cause, severe adrenal exhaustion usually requires hydrocortisone (cortisol) therapy, which consists of small amounts of hydrocortisone taken throughout the day in a pattern that matches your body's natural cortisol production rhythm. You have to have a prescription for hydrocortisone. But first I check a salivary adrenal panel, which is the best test to measure cortisol. I did this, and it worked very well, and like the slow trickle charge for batteries, it slowly recharged my adrenals over a period of several months. Take hydrocortisone with a small amount of food to avoid GI irritation. (I took hydrocortisone along with other adrenal supplements and vitamins, as described earlier in this chapter.)

The good news about your adrenals is that once we restore adrenal function, you can eventually discontinue your hydrocortisone medication. For most people several months of 2.5–5 mg of hydrocortisone medication at mealtimes with 10 mg at breakfast is enough to reboot your system. (I don't recommend prednisone, which is a synthetic glucocorticoid and is four to five times more potent than hydrocortisone and lasts a lot longer, usually twelve hours or longer, because long-term use is associated with many side effects. Bioidentical hydrocortisone provides physiological doses of cortisol, which is the amount your body is supposed to make.) These are small doses, but they work well to get your energy back, increase immune function, decrease inflammation, and help restore your adrenals. All in all, the hydrocortisone helps reset the adrenals. I usually start patients on 10 mg at around 8:00 a.m. with food, 5 mg at noon, 5 mg at 4:00 p.m., and sometimes 2.5–5 mg at bedtime.

Being able to take a medication for a short period of time and then get off of it is appealing to most patients. That certainly applies to the rebooting of your adrenal glands. By contrast, people with adrenal issues who begin taking antianxiety medications often find themselves taking those drugs for life!

THE HORMONE HEALTH ZONE FOR ADRENAL HEALTH

Stress causes a substantial amount of trouble for our bodies and our adrenal glands in particular. When stressors aren't dealt with correctly, symptoms eventually begin to appear. Remember the crazy stat that 75–90 percent of doctor visits are stress related?[3] Well, as we age, our hormones usually decrease to borderline low or low levels, which only compounds the effects of stress all the more.

One very encouraging factor in your adrenal health is that when you optimize your hormone levels, it is usually enough to reboot your adrenal glands as well! The hormone health zone for your adrenals is connected directly to your thyroid and testosterone hormone levels. Because cortisol from the adrenals constantly chips away at your thyroid and testosterone, recharging your adrenal glands automatically is a huge boost to your testosterone and thyroid levels. In essence, you positively impact three hormones for the price of one.

And believe me, when you optimize your testosterone and thyroid and reboot your adrenals, you usually feel incredible. Most of the many negative symptoms we have listed so far are directly impacted by these three hormones, so when you fix these three hormones, you are potentially fixing the lists of symptoms along with them.

When it comes to optimizing your hormone levels and healing your adrenals, let me give you two secrets: (1) for many men and women, optimizing testosterone levels usually improves or resolves adrenal issues, even many times without having to take hydrocortisone, and (2) for women, taking bioidentical micronized progesterone at night usually helps them sleep like a baby. It also helps them grow beautiful hair, decreases irritability, gives a deep sense of calm, and is the answer for any woman with PMS. Clearly, optimizing hormone levels is good across the board, especially if your adrenals need to be recharged.

The more you learn to get in God's rhythm and slow down to rest, the more your body can heal. Even Jesus didn't get in a hurry. When Lazarus was dying, Jesus did not rush there, and because He didn't hurry, we saw His resurrection power. Make it a habit to live in a place of peace and get in His rhythm. For more information on overcoming stress and adrenal fatigue, refer to my book *Stress Less*.

CHAPTER 10

TESTOSTERONE ANSWERS FOR WOMEN

Becky was only forty-eight, but when she called, she complained, "I feel as if I'm ninety-eight!" She flew in from out of state looking for answers. Two years earlier she had had a hysterectomy that included her ovaries, and from that moment forward her body seemed out of order. Her list of symptoms would have scared any woman:

- deep depression
- suicidal tendencies
- lack of sex drive
- bad hot flashes
- dryness and irritation of the vagina
- irritability and grumpiness
- frequent migraines

Her doctor had given her a vaginal estrogen cream, which helped a little with dryness, but it did nothing to help with her other symptoms. He also gave her an antidepressant and gradually kept increasing the dosage. All that seemed to do was make her other symptoms even worse. Her friends, husband, and other family members were almost as upset and frantic for answers as she was.

We checked her hormone levels. Her follicle-stimulating hormone (FSH) number was around 150 IU/L and should have been less than 23 IU/L! (By way of comparison, a young woman in mid-cycle has an FSH of 4.5–23 IU/L.) It was even worse when we checked her estradiol, total testosterone, free testosterone, and progesterone levels. Using a metaphor, she was basically driving her car with no gas in the tank, no oil in the motor, and no air in the tires. No wonder she felt so horrible!

With her depression and history of migraines, she started on a medium dose of testosterone and estradiol (one of the three estrogen hormones), all in pellet form, as that was her preference. Also, she took a natural desiccated thyroid in a sublingual tab.

IT'S A FACT

During their reproductive years, young women usually have three times more testosterone in their bodies than estrogen.

Because she had no uterus, there was no need for progesterone, but she could not sleep. Progesterone is great for helping women sleep, so we gave her a medium dose of bioidentical micronized progesterone at night. She was not overweight, but she went on an anti-inflammatory diet, cutting out gluten and sugar in particular.

Within a week the husband called me. "My wife is back!" he exclaimed. "I really thought I had lost her forever. She is sleeping and has energy, no headaches, vitality, sex drive, and we are a family again. She's not negative or depressed. Thank you!"

A few months later she weaned off her antidepressants as well under the direction of her family physician. In reality it was just her hormone levels. They had crashed as a result of her hysterectomy and removal of her ovaries. (Testosterone in women is primarily produced in the ovaries but also in the adrenal glands and some other tissues.) She was virtually on empty across the board on her hormones. All I did was bring them back up to the optimal level, and she had her life back.

The Three Hormone Dominoes in Women

I have found that women over forty who have had their ovaries removed or who went through menopause before age forty almost always have very low testosterone. That was very much the case with Becky. However, women lose testosterone whether or not they have a hysterectomy. It is in fact usually the first hormone to fall. Here is the bad hormone news for women at a glance:

First hormone domino—Around age forty the levels of testosterone in most women begin to decline.

Second hormone domino—A mere five to ten years later progesterone begins to decline.

Third hormone domino—And five short years after that estradiol starts to decline.

There you have it, the hormone dominoes. The process might be gradual, but it is relentless. The decline can be accelerated by stress, medications, chronic illness, endocrine disruptors, menopause, or removal of the ovaries.

Once the dominoes begin to fall, there is nothing you can do that will sufficiently prop them back up without bioidentical hormone replacement. There is no diet or weight loss program, no pill or drink that will get your curves back, reverse wrinkling, wash away the cellulite, or control the host of other negative symptoms.

It's called "aging" by most people, including many doctors, and women are told to accept the sagging features, the expanding waistlines, and less muscle tone because "that's what happens when you get older." Even the irritability, lack of libido, and depression are included in the package and are usually treated with medication, especially antidepressants. Let's look at each domino a little more closely.

Domino 1: testosterone

Testosterone is the first domino to fall. Though essential for women's hormone balance, around age forty it usually starts to decline rapidly. (At age forty, women usually have half the testosterone they had at twenty.) It is part of the woman's natural shift from a reproductive to nonreproductive stage of life, but still, it's no fun!

Domino 2: progesterone

Then five to ten years later, at approximately age forty-five, progesterone levels begin to lower as women hit menopause and their ovaries hit or miss with progesterone production. When progesterone starts to decline, a host of ailments come right with it, including:

- heavy bleeding
- breast enlargement
- breast tenderness
- bloating
- poor sleep
- moodiness
- PMS
- joint pain
- fatigue
- water retention
- cholesterol rises

As the progesterone peters out, the only hormone left is estrogen.

Domino 3: estrogen (estradiol)

At this point, approximately five years later (typically between ages fifty and fifty-five), testosterone is usually so low that it has virtually no impact on the woman's body. If stress and medications are also in the system (e.g., antidepressants, cholesterol-lowering drugs, antianxiety drugs, insomnia drugs, and so on), then you can forget about testosterone. It's usually gone.

With progesterone also on a steep decline, there is one hormone left that seeks to rule the woman's body: estrogen. That might not sound very bad, since estrogen is known as the female hormone, but there are three main types of estrogen, and it's not the good type of estrogen that wins the battle. Estrogen comes in three main forms:

E1 (estrone): This hormone fights to dominate as soon as progesterone levels begin to decrease. This is the "old lady estrogen," or, as I prefer to call it, the "elderly estrogen," and is the main estrogen in the female after menopause. It characteristically causes muscle to be replaced with fat (especially in the belly and back), raises bad cholesterol, increases the risk for breast cancer and heart disease, and contributes to sagging and painful breasts, sagging skin, obesity, irritability, and poor memory.

E2 (estradiol): This hormone was dominant in your childbearing years. It is the preferred estrogen because it is responsible for women's curves, round hips, perky breasts, moist vagina, higher metabolism, muscle tone, elasticity of the skin and vagina, soft and supple skin, thick and shiny hair, happier mood, and stronger memory.

E3 (estriol): This hormone is always a minor player, but its characteristics are more like estradiol than estrone. It does not cause breast cancer, but it is weaker than estrone and cannot dominate in the estrogen power play. It comes from the placenta and is a pregnancy estrogen that increases the storage of fat for breast-feeding.[1]

There you have it, the estrogen battle that is waged in every woman's body. Eventually estrone will rule. It always does.

THE ANSWER TO CELLULITE

Low oxygen levels cause a pocket or dimple in the skin. The skin needs more oxygen and greater blood flow, and the answer is more testosterone. Optimized testosterone levels reduce and sometimes totally remove cellulite.

Estradiol, the pretty and youthful estrogen, the estrogen that all women want, will fight valiantly for a decade or more, but with no support from testosterone or progesterone, and constant internal attacks from stress, medications, endocrine disruptors, poor nutrition, a lack of exercise, and more, it will inevitably give way to estrone.

And estrone will rule with an iron fist! It is merciless. If you thought the loss of progesterone brought with it a wave of unpleasant symptoms, estrone dominance is far worse. Common symptoms I see every day include:

- wrinkles
- cellulite
- anxiety
- saggy breasts and skin
- thin skin
- hair loss
- insomnia
- belly fat
- hot flashes
- dry vagina
- recurrent UTIs
- poor memory

- almost an aversion to sex
- increased risk of breast cancer (one in eight women)
- dry skin
- painful breasts

- irritability
- chin hair
- slowing metabolism
- muscle shrinkage and replacement with fat

You are no doubt wondering if there is any good news. Yes, there is! Dominoes that have fallen can be righted again. For that matter, they didn't need to fall in the first place! This means you can get your body back! You can get your health back! You can get your dreams back! I have found with optimized levels of estradiol and testosterone, you can keep your healthy-looking body into old age, and that includes all the benefits associated with it.

The negative symptoms you dislike so much can usually be reversed and many times completely eliminated. So the next time you hear, "Well, that's what happens as you age," you can breathe a sigh of relief because it doesn't apply to you!

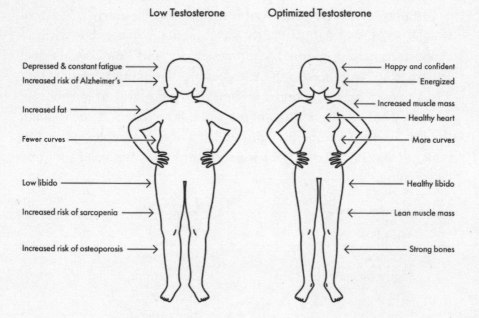

Low Testosterone

Optimized Testosterone

Depressed & constant fatigue →
Increased risk of Alzheimer's →

Increased fat →

Fewer curves →

Low libido →

Increased risk of sarcopenia →

Increased risk of osteoporosis →

← Happy and confident
← Energized

← Increased muscle mass
← Healthy heart

← More curves

← Healthy libido

← Lean muscle mass

← Strong bones

TESTOSTERONE IN WOMEN

The first hormone women need to optimize is testosterone. Although women produce a lot less testosterone than men (about 10 percent of what men produce), having sufficient testosterone in our bodies is equally essential for everyone.[2] After all, testosterone "is the central hormone in the aging process."[3] It may sound a little strange to recommend testosterone therapy for women, but with it they can:

- slow, stop, or sometimes reverse cellulite
- lose weight, especially belly fat
- recharge the metabolism
- tighten skin
- wash away irritability
- boost energy levels
- feel empowered
- build muscle
- improve wrinkles
- restore libido
- improve memory
- vanquish night sweats
- decrease inflammation
- strengthen the heart
- improve and sometimes stop a leaky bladder
- prevent bladder infections

Accomplishing this list is amazing enough, but there is more good news about the benefits of testosterone, including:

- "The genetically predetermined onset of Alzheimer's...can be delayed ten years by replacing testosterone prior to menopause. When estradiol is added at menopause, there is an additional ten-year delay in the onset of dementia or Alzheimer's."[4]

- Low testosterone is linked to an increased risk of diabetes, hardening of the arteries, and weak bones.[5]

- Low testosterone increases your chances of elevated total cholesterol, LDL cholesterol, and triglycerides and decreased growth hormone.[6]

- The lack of interest in sex is primarily from low testosterone, depression, and medications.[7]

- Testosterone helps reboot the adrenals.

- Bioidentical testosterone pellets plus Arimidex help prevent recurrent breast cancer.[8]

- Testosterone improves energy, concentration, stamina, and mood.

- Testosterone helps rebuild bone. (Osteoporosis affects women over men 4 to 1.)

You may have noticed that low testosterone levels give women many of the symptoms associated with hypothyroidism. This serves as another strong motivator for women to keep their testosterone levels up.

TESTOSTERONE IN REAL LIFE

For years I have told couples not to get divorced until they both get their hormones checked, balanced, and optimized. Every marriage counselor, family counselor, psychologist, and pastor should know this!

TESTOSTERONE-KILLING DRUGS FOR WOMEN

1. Antidepressants

2. Cholesterol-lowering drugs

3. BP-lowering drugs, especially beta-blockers and Aldactone

4. Birth control pills

5. Oral estrogens

What typically happens is that the woman hits age forty, and her sex drive drops dramatically. (Remember what happens to her testosterone domino at that age?) Then, about ten unsatisfying years later, surrounded by stress and drama, the man turns fifty, and he suddenly has erectile dysfunction issues. (The same low testosterone is now affecting the man, just ten years later.)

What to do? Most often the man goes and gets a prescription to handle his ED issues, a pill that has a list of adverse side effects, but he is willing to put up with them for the sake of his manliness. A growing number of men will get testosterone replacement therapy, and that boosts their sex drive as well as muscle growth, weight loss, vitality, and energy.

So now the man is pumped and attracted to his wife...but she won't touch him. Is the man willing to put up with another ten long, sad years? Not likely.

Years ago I had a husband and wife (their combined age equaled 140 years) stop in at my office who wanted to optimize their hormone levels at the same time. A few weeks later they called to say they felt as if they were on their honeymoon again. All we did was optimize their hormone levels, but it was their improved testosterone levels that caused the biggest impact. For marriages, that is incredible news! (I have seen hundreds of marriages restored after they both got their testosterone levels back on track.)

Most often it is the man who boosts his testosterone levels alone, but it can happen to women as well. Usually once they get their hormone levels optimized, their curves start to come back, and they have boundless energy, feel great, and are loving life again. But the husband is an overweight slug on the couch! (Obesity lowers testosterone all the more.)

Believe it or not, many of the troubles we face in marriage are the result of our testosterone levels going lower and lower. This is obviously not all about sex; this is about life, marriage, family, fun, health, and being all that we were meant to be. How can we bring glory and honor to God when our lives are falling apart?

Of course hormone levels are not the answer to everything, but they do play an important part in every area of life. Testosterone's effect on our lives starts in our brain, more so than we often think. Here are three key ways it works in the brain.

1. Testosterone turn-on

Testosterone is responsible for what gives us the interest and desire for sex. Believe it or not, the brain is the most sexual organ of all. And testosterone makes the brain aware of sexual touch, gives sexual climax, and basically makes it happen. Take away testosterone, and we are all duds, with no interest at all.

When women are young, testosterone suppresses estrone, but when testosterone is gone, estrone increases, and the loss of libido is a direct result. The return of libido is one of the first signs that testosterone therapy is working.

IT'S A FACT

"Couples who have a healthy sex life live longer and report more satisfaction in their lives than those who do not."[9]

Antidepressants are a big turnoff because they usually lower testosterone levels even further, but testosterone is, in my opinion, the best antidepressant on the market, and it turns the brain on.

Not long ago a couple who had been married for more than thirty years came to see me. He had recently had a heart attack and bypass surgery. He was not the strongest man out there, but he wanted his life and wife back. She had no interest in sex at all. Three months later they were back for a checkup. She spoke up, "In all honesty, we were lucky to have sex once every two weeks, but now we are three times a week, and it's not just boring. It's exciting. We love it."

She would have called me a liar if I had told her before we started the testosterone therapy that she might say that, but that is the power of testosterone. It can turn things on that have been off for a long time.

Another woman, age seventy-five, was overjoyed to experience a sexual climax again—she hadn't had one in more than twenty years—but that is one side effect of optimizing testosterone levels.

2. Testosterone tune-in

As we have already mentioned, Alzheimer's can be delayed ten years by replacing testosterone prior to menopause, and if you add estradiol, you get an additional ten-year delay in the onset of dementia or Alzheimer's.[10] In fact, scientists are exploring the notion that Alzheimer's can be prevented by optimizing testosterone levels.[11]

That is absolutely incredible! Testosterone can tune in your brain like nothing else. Anyone suffering from memory-related illnesses or trying to avoid them due to a family history needs to optimize his or her testosterone levels as quickly as possible.

My dad spent twelve years warehoused in a nursing home. Nothing could help, and he slowly wasted away. That is not what you or I want to experience.

Memory-related diseases affect women more than men, one result I believe to be the result of men having more testosterone in their bodies for a longer period of time than women. By optimizing testosterone levels, along with following an anti-inflammatory diet, moderate exercise, a healthy lifestyle, good sleep, less stress, and so on, women are maximizing their brain health and strength. That is a smart move!

Without testosterone and estradiol,[12] the brain eventually shrinks! It really does. But the same hormones also repair brain neurons, increase neurotransmitter production, decrease inflammation, increase blood flow and oxygen, and improve the overall thought process. And adding these hormones can delay Alzheimer's by twenty years. If that isn't a good enough reason to optimize your hormone levels, I don't know what is!

3. Testosterone take-on

Remember when you were younger, and you wanted to live forever, dream huge dreams, and take life by the horns? Did that just disappear because you got older, started a career, and became responsible? I don't think so. My belief is that many of us have lost hope, inspiration, and excitement for the future because our testosterone levels have dropped precipitously low.

IT'S A FACT

Every gland that produces wetness dries out when testosterone levels are low, especially the eyes.[13]

When hormone levels are optimized to what they were when we were twenty years old, depression and anxiety usually lift. (Like I said, testosterone is the best antidepressant out there, and it beats anxiety as well.) What is more, we have improved mood, increased optimism, and more belief in self. This is not a mind game. Nobody is psyching you out. This is real, internal belief and positive mood that come from elevated testosterone levels.

Optimizing your testosterone levels will result in better strength and stamina, enhanced mood and well-being, more energy and motivation, improved skin tone and collagen, greater protection against heart attack and stroke, lower blood pressure, lessened arthritis pain, boosted immune function, better wound healing, and stronger tendons, ligaments, and joints.[14]

How will you feel when this describes you? Yes, you too will feel you can take on the world. And feeling like that, you could!

How Is Your Testosterone Level?

You know how the hormone dominoes fall for women, and you see the many benefits of testosterone, but do you know your testosterone levels? I have collected a short list of low-testosterone signals that may help you gauge your own testosterone levels. Blood work is needed to confirm suspicions, but persistent symptoms are hard to argue away.

When patients tell me how they feel and rattle off this list of items, they are usually low in testosterone. How about you? Do these words describe you?

- tiredness ("bone tired") often
- inability to sleep at night
- inability to feel rested in the morning
- depression
- weight gain (especially belly fat)
- lack of or little sex drive
- more common migraines
- irritability and grumpiness
- weaker muscles
- lack of sexual climax
- brain fog
- aching joints
- thin skin with increased wrinkles
- lack of zest for life

There are many more symptoms I could read, but most of you were probably already nodding in agreement by the time you read just halfway through the list. Low testosterone is the cause, and the great news is, it's fixable!

THE HORMONE HEALTH ZONE FOR TESTOSTERONE IN WOMEN

Few women know that they have quite a bit of testosterone in their bodies, primarily when they are young. In their twenties and thirties their testosterone is in the normal range. After forty is when we start to see the decline.

And if you are in range, that is great. However, as we have discussed, there are numerous factors that push testosterone levels lower and lower (aging, removal of ovaries, menopause, medications, stress, and more). If you find yourself at the lower end of these ranges, or even below them, your body is crying out for more testosterone.

SIDE EFFECTS

There are usually no negative side effects from raising testosterone levels in women. Countless symptoms are lessened or removed by raising testosterone levels.

Sadly most doctors are taught to prescribe only low doses of estradiol (in pill format, which is not good) and no testosterone whatsoever! In fact, doctors usually choose not to address hormone issues at all! They will tell you the "normal ranges" (you will probably be in range), and if you happen to be low, they will usually prescribe you a medication for the symptoms.

That will never get your health back. What your body needs is bioidentical hormone therapy. You may need to find another doctor, someone who will treat your low-testosterone symptoms with bioidentical testosterone.

I have found boosting testosterone levels with pellets to be very effective and efficient. They raise levels quickly, and you don't need to come back for another treatment for three to four months and sometimes six months. Testosterone injections are the next-best method if pellets are too pricey, followed by testosterone creams. Injections are usually given one or two times a week. Testosterone cream can be put behind one knee every day or directly on the female sex organ every other day or three times each week. For some women, I have also used a sublingual testosterone tab compounded at a compounding pharmacy.

With pellets, women can get their total testosterone levels up to around 60–70 ng/dL within one week! After that, maintaining testosterone levels around 60–70 ng/dL is ideal for most women and sometimes even higher. They feel amazing, bone growth happens, fat is replaced with muscle, the brain is energized, the heart is stronger, and energy levels increase rapidly.

As for free testosterone, doctors (especially endocrinologists) will recommend very low levels according to your age, such as 0.2–5.0 pg/mL for those ages eighteen through sixty-nine and 0.3–5.0 pg/mL for women ages seventy through eighty-nine. Women whose numbers match their recommendations usually also have matching low-testosterone symptoms! The recommended normal ranges for total testosterone and free testosterone in women are as follows:

Total testosterone: 2.0–45 ng/dL

Free testosterone: 0.2–5.0 pg/mL

When your testosterone levels are optimized (pushed to the upper ranges or a little higher) to the levels you were at when you were in your twenties, your numbers will be closer to these:

Total testosterone: 60–70 ng/dL (higher for those with osteoporosis or sarcopenia)

Free testosterone: 5–10 pg/mL

At these optimized levels amazing things happen. For my female patients with sarcopenia (feebleness) and osteoporosis, I may get their total testosterone level as high as 150–200 ng/dL, which helps reverse sarcopenia and osteoporosis in many of them. I believe testosterone replacement is the best way to overcome osteoporosis with rarely having side effects, unlike most of the medications that treat osteoporosis.

It's Your Decision

Each woman has her own wants and needs. How about you? Perhaps one of these desires matches that of your own:

- Want to boost your metabolism?
- Need to increase your stamina and energy?
- Wish brain fog would go away for good?
- Want your lean body back?
- Want to improve your immune system?
- Need depression to lift forever?
- Want help with your memory?
- Want strong bones (even reverse osteoporosis and osteopenia)?
- Want to lower cholesterol?
- Need arthritis pains improved or relieved?
- Want to reset your adrenals?
- Wish for restored libido and sexual climax?
- Want to protect your brain?
- Need protection against breast cancer?
- Want to prevent, improve, and sometimes stop a leaky bladder and bladder infections?
- Want to lose weight?

One hormone can meet all these requests! Testosterone is that answer, at optimized levels.

I suggest women in their forties start monitoring their testosterone levels. The time to start optimizing testosterone levels is when the hormone levels go below 50–60 percent of upper range or when symptoms develop. Below 50 percent most people begin to develop persistent low-testosterone symptoms. You know your body, so you track it as you go.

When your testosterone levels are optimized, life is great! Psalm 40:2–3 captures the transformation many women achieve when they break free from the symptoms that have plagued them for years:

> He also brought me up out of a horrible pit, out of the miry clay, and set my feet upon a rock, and established my steps. *He has put a new song in my mouth"* (emphasis added).

That's the way it's supposed to be.

CHAPTER 11

PROGESTERONE ANSWERS FOR WOMEN

C HRONIC ILLNESS IS often one of the most difficult things we face in life. By its nature it is constant, often painful, not flattering, expensive, and inescapable. Like any doctor, I want to be able to help people dealing with chronic illness. With bioidentical hormone therapy, that is possible.

Several years ago Winona visited my office. She had suffered from fibromyalgia for a long time and was looking for some relief. She was not my first fibromyalgia patient, and I could tell she was in a lot of pain. She was still funny, almost comedic, but her true personality was being held back by her sickness.

"When was the last time someone hugged you?" I asked. Her answer broke my heart.

"It's been more than twenty-five years," she replied matter-of-factly.

I couldn't believe it. Imagine no hugs or touches, no grandkids with their arms around your neck, and not much intimacy with anyone for twenty-five years! She was starved for love, but with pain throughout the body, an aversion to pressure, and a heightened sensitivity to touch and pain, it didn't look as if much would change. In many ways it was as if she suffered from modern-day leprosy.

"What is it that you want the most?" I probed.

"I can't sleep very well, and I desperately want to be able to sleep," she stated. "When I do eventually fall asleep, it's almost time to get up for the day, and I wake up already exhausted."

Looking at her chart, I knew exactly why she could not sleep. Her progesterone was less than 0.5 ng/mL—extremely low compared with the recommended 10–20 ng/mL for optimized progesterone levels. Adding her low progesterone numbers to the adrenal fatigue and insomnia she had as a result of fibromyalgia, which usually was associated with high cortisol levels at night, she could forget about sleep. It wasn't happening.

"Irritable?" I asked with a smile.

"Come closer, and I'll bite you!" she laughed.

Women with PMS are irritable because they are usually low in progesterone, but the same is usually true for women without PMS who are low in progesterone. I have found that micronized progesterone is the *best* treatment for PMS.

"How about anxious?" I questioned.

"All the time," she answered.

"Depressed?" I asked.

"Of course," she replied. "What else would you expect?"

Progesterone binds to receptors in the brain to help calm us down and give us a sense of peace, but if progesterone levels are low, that certainly wouldn't be happening.

Despite her valiant effort to stay upbeat, she was really hurting.

"Admit it," she joked. "I'm a train wreck."

Her treatment began with moderate doses of bioidentical micronized progesterone at bedtime. She absolutely had to start sleeping well. We also worked to get her other hormones optimized, especially her thyroid. (Almost all fibromyalgia patients have low free T3 levels and low testosterone levels.) Her adrenal glands were extremely fatigued from the chronic illness, and she had low cortisol levels, so we worked to reboot those as well with hydrocortisone. We also dealt with some pent-up emotions, traumas, and unforgiveness and then put her on an anti-inflammatory diet.

IT'S A FACT

Progesterone levels decrease in all women when they are premenstrual.

She was willing to do whatever it took to get free of the symptoms that had been dragging her down for decades. A few short months later Winona was back for a checkup. When she walked into the room, I stood to greet her, and she walked right up to me and gave me a big hug!

I was shocked. But then I was so glad for her. The twenty-five years of pain on the outside, while aching on the inside for touch, was finally gone! It was incredible. And she truly looked happy.

"I'm back!" she exclaimed, and I knew what she meant.

And that is simply the power of bioidentical hormones at work in our bodies.

PROGESTERONE—THE SECOND HORMONE TO FALL

In women you remember that progesterone is the second hormone domino to fall. It typically happens just five to ten years after testosterone has started its rapid decline.

Renowned board-certified OB-GYN specialist Gary Donovitz states that by age forty a woman's progesterone production may have decreased by 80 percent.[1] That is a massive drop! To be left with a mere 20 percent of what is normal is never going to be enough to meet life's demands.

When women's bodies are not making enough progesterone, the symptoms of low progesterone are going to naturally appear. Those negative side effects or symptoms will be something like those in the following chart, which you can rate for yourself.

SYMPTOM	RATE IT			
	0 (NEVER)	1 (OCCASIONALLY)	2 (OFTEN)	3 (ALWAYS)
Bloating	0	1	2	3
Breast tenderness	0	1	2	3
Depression	0	1	2	3
Feelings of anxiety	0	1	2	3
Fluid retention	0	1	2	3
Food cravings	0	1	2	3
Grumpiness	0	1	2	3
Headaches	0	1	2	3
Insomnia	0	1	2	3
Irritability	0	1	2	3
Miscarriages	0	1	2	3
Mood swings	0	1	2	3
Muscle aches	0	1	2	3
PMS	0	1	2	3

SYMPTOM	RATE IT			
	0 (NEVER)	1 (OCCASIONALLY)	2 (OFTEN)	3 (ALWAYS)
Swelling	0	1	2	3
Thinning hair	0	1	2	3
UTIs	0	1	2	3

These symptoms are begging for answers. Unfortunately prescription drugs can often patch the problem, temporarily alleviating a symptom, but the core issue of low progesterone hormone levels is not addressed. What happens? More symptoms often appear, and usually with greater severity. Then it's a "train wreck," just as Winona said.

CONFUSION STILL SURROUNDS PROGESTERONE

Like every hormone, there are myths and fears that swirl around progesterone. But like with the other hormones, more and more studies are being done to find the truth, the real value, behind progesterone. That includes everything from type (bioidentical versus synthetic) to dosage and lasting effects. Bioidentical, micronized progesterone protects women against breast cancer; however, synthetic progestin (the synthetic counterfeit for bioidentical, micronized progesterone) increases one's risk of breast cancer.

Here is a little recap about progesterone that will help clarify some of the confusion out there:

Breast cell growth: It is synthetic progestin that stimulates breast cell growth, not bioidentical, micronized progesterone, which has a protective effect.[2]

Increased breast cancer risk: Bioidentical, micronized progesterone is not associated with an increase in breast cancer risk.[3]

Breast cancer: Many studies have shown an increased risk of breast cancer when synthetic progestins are used.[4]

Protection from breast cancer: Bioidentical progesterone protects women against breast cancer.[5]

Cardiovascular risk: Synthetic progestin reduces good (HDL) cholesterol levels in women.[6]

Even with all this, and countless many more studies from around the world, many doctors still prescribe synthetic progestins, and many are still afraid to prescribe bioidentical progesterone to women who are ten years past menopause out of fear of causing heart attacks, cancer, blood clots, or another problem. Bioidentical progesterone does not increase the risk, but they are still hesitant.

I warn patients who have a primary care doctor or ob-gyn who prescribes them a synthetic prescription for progesterone: "Do not take it. You are increasing your risks for breast cancer, heart attacks, strokes, blood clots, and more. If the progesterone is not micronized and bioidentical, do not fill your prescription." That is how serious this is, but as always patients make their own choices.

Doctors and patients need to remember that optimizing hormones is only returning those hormones to the upper range of normal. That should not scare anyone away.

IT'S A FACT

What is the average age of menopause in the United States? Age 51.[7]

Do All Women Need Progesterone?

Women with a uterus need progesterone because progesterone protects the uterus from abnormal bleeding and from developing uterine cancer, especially when women are on estrogen replacement. But what if a woman has had a hysterectomy or gone through menopause? That's a fair question, but I answer that with, "Do women want to sleep better, reduce depression and irritability, have thick, beautiful hair, and minimize mood swings?" The need for progesterone does not disappear, whatever a woman's season of life.

For women who have had trouble getting pregnant or have had miscarriages, they definitely need to watch their progesterone levels. Progesterone helps them become and stay pregnant. It also helps protect the uterus during pregnancy. When women complain about infertility, I not only check their progesterone levels; I also check their thyroid levels. A sluggish thyroid is a sure way of keeping a woman from getting pregnant.

If women have too little progesterone, they often have too much estrogen and usually are estrogen dominant, and as a result they are usually emotional, irritable, anxious, and edgy. This is very common around age fifty when the second hormone domino (progesterone) falls. When progesterone levels are optimized (along with estrogen, thyroid, and testosterone levels, since you want to optimize all the hormones at once), the body is usually calmer and not ruled by the emotional side of the often-dominating estrogen hormone.

Three of the most common symptoms of women who are low in progesterone are irritability, an inability to sleep well at night, and PMS. And whether or not they have had a hysterectomy, optimizing their progesterone levels usually helps alleviate all these symptoms. We are not talking about "patching" anything; we are talking about fixing it permanently, and that usually happens. With optimized progesterone levels, I've found these symptoms rarely return, and women love that!

The Hormone Health Zone for Progesterone in Women

According to LabCorp, the ranges for women's progesterone hormone levels fluctuate a lot. Consider these numbers:[8]

follicular phase: 0.1–0.9 ng/mL

luteal phase: 1.8–23.9 ng/mL

ovulatory phase: 0.1–12.0 ng/mL

And if pregnant, those numbers change even more:

first trimester: 11.0–44.3 ng/mL

second trimester: 25.4–83.3 ng/mL

third trimester: 58.7–214.0 ng/mL

And if postmenopausal:

0.0–0.1 ng/mL

Interestingly a man's progesterone level is virtually nothing, down at 0.0–0.5 ng/mL. Any more than that, and he will experience symptoms similar to low testosterone, principally a significant decrease in sex drive, if he takes progesterone. So men should never take progesterone in pill or cream form!

An extremely low level is fine for a man, but no woman usually wants to live at that level! Winona, the woman whose story I shared at the start of this chapter, had progesterone levels as low as those of a man, and that was one of the reasons she felt the way she did and suffered from insomnia.

So if you are postmenopausal or have had a hysterectomy, what is the optimum progesterone level? The goal for optimized hormone levels is to mirror your levels when you were in your twenties. At that time 10–20 ng/mL was your normal upper range, and that is the range we aim for again.

The recommended normal ranges for progesterone in women are as follows:

progesterone as adult: 0.1–25 ng/mL

progesterone when pregnant: 10–290 ng/mL

progesterone when postmenopausal: 0.1–1.0 ng/mL

For pregnant women, keeping progesterone levels high enough to maintain the pregnancy is the goal. For women pre and postmenopausal, their optimized progesterone levels should be closer to these:

progesterone as an adult: 10–20 ng/mL

progesterone when postmenopausal: 10–20 ng/mL

Most women who need progesterone therapy usually fall in the postmenopausal category, so returning their progesterone levels to 10–20 ng/mL is exactly what the body needs.

How is it applied—with pills, sublingual tabs, or creams? For bioidentical progesterone, one of the best methods is with sublingual tabs under the tongue before bedtime. The sublingual tabs are easy to use, are inexpensive, are very effective, and come in varying dosages.

The same method works for women who are trying to get pregnant. Approximate sublingual or oral dosages are:

- raising progesterone hormone levels toward optimization: 75–300 mg at bedtime; I start women over 65 at lower dosages such as 75 mg and monitor progesterone levels

- raising progesterone hormone levels to aid in getting pregnant: 50–75 mg daily and sometimes more

Taking sublingual tabs of bioidentical progesterone before bed will usually make you sleepy. If you are a woman battling depression or fighting a chronic illness, this is perfect! A good night's sleep is vital.

The micronized progesterone is created from plants, and it matches the progesterone in a woman's body. As expected, synthetic progesterone does not and causes the many bad side effects already mentioned. Bioidentical progesterone therapy is one of the most powerful health tools available. That means feeling miserable for the rest of your life is no longer an option.

CHAPTER 12

ESTROGEN ANSWERS FOR WOMEN

HIT A WALL," LuAnn said. "My body no longer obeys me. I go on a diet; no change. I quit eating gluten; no change. I exercise more; no change. I go to the gym; no change. I'm tempted to quit eating, but I don't even think that will work either."

She was evidently discouraged.

"What is the problem?" I asked, trying to figure out what ailed her the most. Her charts were pretty bare without much blood work done in the past few years.

"Basically, I feel like a brick. I used to have an hourglass figure, now I'm stuck with this," she complained, pointing at her waist.

LuAnn had indeed lost her curves, though she was not obese. All her efforts to stay in shape were actually helping, but she was on a gradual slide that could not be stopped by diet and exercise alone.

"My husband and I have all this free time to do whatever we want to do, and I try to exercise, walk, run, jog, bike, even do hot yoga, but nothing helps very much," she lamented.

She was fifty-seven years old, a mother of two grown children, and married to a businessman who retired early. They lived in a great neighborhood near the mountains in North Carolina, but it was obvious she wasn't enjoying it all that much as of late.

"Is your husband pretty fit himself?" I asked.

"He's a little soft around the middle, but whenever he gets serious at the gym for a few months, he tones right up," she explained. "But not me; nothing works for me."

We ran her blood work, and a few days later my suspicions were confirmed. When LuAnn came back for the results, I explained that her body had been taken hostage by the cruel, merciless queen of estrogen: estrone! She didn't understand.

I broke it down for her just as I did for you in chapter 10, explaining that women have three primary estrogens (E1: estrone, E2: estradiol, and E3: estriol) and that the battle raging inside of her was between two very different and competing estrogens. That made sense to her. Then I explained to LuAnn about the three hormone dominoes, which are also covered in chapter 10.

IT'S A FACT

The only known "prevention" for Alzheimer's and dementia is to optimize estradiol and testosterone levels.[1]

I pointed out that when estrone takes over, women often have additional symptoms far beyond the physical ones she was complaining about. (I'll list these symptoms later in this chapter.) "When estradiol falls, estrone takes over, and women tend to age at warp speed from that moment forward," I added.

She understood that and instantly demanded, "So what can I do right now to kick this estrone off the throne?"

THE SLIDE ALL WOMEN RIDE

Like millions of women, LuAnn found herself on the slippery slope of estrogen right at the point where the amount of wanted estrogen (estradiol) dips much lower than the amount of unwanted estrogen (estrone).

Women can feel it. They know something is happening to their bodies, and they can see it in the mirror, but seldom are they healthy one day and sick the next. Because it is a gradual slide, aging is usually blamed. Or they think, "I will go on a diet this summer, and that will fix it."

Eventually, however, as the level of good estradiol lowers and the level of bad estrone increases, more and more symptoms come to the surface, just as I told LuAnn. One by one women begin to notice many of the symptoms in the following chart, which you can rate for yourself.

SYMPTOMS OF GOOD ESTRADIOL LOWERING			
SYMPTOM	RATE IT		
	0 (NEVER)	1 (OCCASIONALLY)	2 (OFTEN)	3 (ALWAYS)
Allergies increasing, regardless of allergy season	0	1	2	3
Clouded thinking	0	1	2	3
Difficulty getting to sleep and staying asleep	0	1	2	3
Dryness everywhere, especially vaginal dryness	0	1	2	3
Energy levels bottoming out	0	1	2	3
Exhaustion upon waking up	0	1	2	3
Headaches	0	1	2	3
Inability to lose weight, especially belly fat	0	1	2	3
Increased anxiety	0	1	2	3
Increased bone loss	0	1	2	3
Increasing facial hair	0	1	2	3
Irritability	0	1	2	3
Loss of curves	0	1	2	3
Memory issues	0	1	2	3
More frequent bladder infections	0	1	2	3
Muscle and joint pain	0	1	2	3
Perky breasts starting to sag	0	1	2	3
Possible irregular heartbeat	0	1	2	3
Sexual climax becoming infrequent	0	1	2	3
Vaginal dryness	0	1	2	3
Wrinkles appearing all over with sagging skin	0	1	2	3

This may be a slide that all women ride, but they also all want to get off of it as soon as possible. Thankfully that can become a reality when they optimize their hormone levels.

WHY DID ESTROGEN TURN AGAINST ME?

For women, it does seem that estrogen has turned against them. Their "young lady" feminine features from one estrogen suddenly in a few short years turned into "elderly lady," not-so-flattering features from another estrogen. What is the deal?

To begin with, the fact that there are three different types of estrogen at work in your body explains a lot. The next factor women must understand is that menopause, simply put, shuts down the ovaries. They stop releasing eggs and stop optimal production of hormones. Consider this:

> Estrogen's perfect harmony: Before women enter menopause, estradiol was mostly made in their ovaries and to a smaller degree in their adrenals, liver, and fatty tissue as well. All the estradiol they need is converted beautifully in their ovaries. Estradiol is the estrogen that makes a woman look youthful and feminine with a slender waistline, perky breasts, soft skin, a moist vagina, a good mood, and thick and shiny hair.

IT'S A FACT

- Menopause is diagnosed once you've gone twelve months without a menstrual period.
- Postmenopause is the season of life following menopause.

Estrogen's nightmare: After women enter menopause, suddenly the ovaries stop producing estradiol. That means very little estrone is converted to estradiol. (If your ovaries have been removed, you have almost a complete and sudden stop of estrone-to-estradiol conversion!) But the other places in the body, such as the liver, adrenals, and fatty tissue, keep on making estrone, but there is hardly any conversion to estradiol taking place anywhere in your body. This leads to all of the unwanted symptoms already listed elsewhere in this book.

There you have it. For the most part, the estrogen you want (estradiol) basically stops being produced after menopause. You may still have a very small amount of estradiol being converted in other parts of the body, but it is never at the same level as before menopause.

Remember the story of Sarah in the Bible? She was well past her childbearing years. Estrone was probably the dominant estrogen in her body, but she probably still had some estradiol since she was elderly and still beautiful. The chances of her getting pregnant were zero—until God intervened!

You see, when women are young, they have a 2-to-1 ratio of estradiol to estrone. Your body loves it, but that 2-to-1 ratio is usually ruined at or after menopause. And when the final hormone domino of estrogen falls, that ratio is never going to be achieved again on its own. It's over!

But you can get your body restored to its ideal 2-to-1 ratio! You can start reversing the aging process! And the answer might surprise you.

The Hormone Health Zone for Estrogen in Women

Optimizing your estrogen hormone levels focuses not on boosting your estradiol (E2) levels to the 2-to-1 ratio over estrone (E1) but on lowering your follicle-stimulating hormone (FSH) levels to less than 23 IU/L (international units per milliliter). Let me explain.

Estradiol can be like a double-edged sword for some women. High normal estradiol levels can cause dysfunctional uterine bleeding; heavy, painful periods; severe menstrual cramps; fibrocystic breast disease; and the return of periods in postmenopausal women. It also fuels most gynecological problems, including uterine fibroids, endometriosis, and some female cancers. For these reasons I do not optimize estrogen levels in women, and some women should even avoid estrogens (such as women with breast, ovarian, or uterine cancer). Women with endometriosis and fibroids require much smaller amounts of estradiol so that it doesn't reactivate their disease.

I can usually help women avoid most or all of the above symptoms by focusing on the FSH, which is a pituitary hormone. When a woman's FSH level is greater than 23 IU/L on two separate blood tests two weeks apart, then they are menopausal and no longer fertile. They can stop birth control pills without fear of getting pregnant. After menopause, my goal is to give enough estradiol to suppress the FSH level to below 23 IU/L. I find that estradiol pellets usually work the best at getting FSH levels to 23 or less.

When the FSH is less than 23, usually most all the main symptoms of menopause are resolved, including vaginal dryness, hot flashes, night sweats, painful intercourse, poor sleep, and mood disturbances. Hot flashes and night sweats are usually caused by a surge of FSH, which triggers the sympathetic nervous system to release adrenaline, which in turn causes the stress response to be stimulated with an increased heart rate.

SIDE EFFECTS

- **What about periods?** Women do not want to have a period again, and bioidentical hormone replacement therapy in pellet form may cause some women to have a period again. **The answer:** If women want estradiol pellets, increasing progesterone levels will stop the bleeding over 90 percent of the time. Some women may need to use a bioidentical estradiol and estriol cream (such as Biest) or transdermal patch instead of pellets to prevent bleeding.

- **What about breast cancer?** Bioidentical hormones do not cause breast cancer. Online sources will tell you that, but it is not true. The Women's Health Initiative proved a 23–33 percent decrease in breast cancer in women taking estrogen only.[2] But if women have breast cancer, I would not recommend estradiol pellets or any estrogen, for that matter. **The answer:** Testosterone pellets are fine, and I recommend taking them with an aromatase inhibitor (such as Arimidex) to keep testosterone from aromatizing to estrogen. Once cancer is in remission, I may prescribe estriol vaginal cream to be applied one to two times a week. I also recommend that women get a mammogram every one to two years.

- **What about fibroids, endometriosis, blood clots, or pelvic pain?** Estradiol is not the cause but may make these conditions worse. **The answer:** Use lower dosages of estradiol pellets or a lower dosage of bioidentical estradiol/estriol cream (such as Biest) or patches or estradiol vaginal cream. Also consider using estriol 0.3 percent cream applied to the labia and vagina once or twice a week. This is the weakest estrogen and is less likely to fuel these conditions.

There is another part of the optimizing estrogen process that you must account for as well. When women hit menopause and the tug of war between estrone and estradiol begins, something happens behind the scenes that does not get as much attention. Two pituitary hormones essential for reproduction, follicle-stimulating hormone (FSH) and luteinizing hormone (LH), begin to increase with no opposition. The less estradiol in your system, the higher these two (especially LH) will climb, and usually the higher they go, the more brain degeneration you might experience.[3]

That's right! Keeping these two hormones in check by optimizing your hormone levels (especially estradiol and testosterone) may help prevent Alzheimer's and dementia.[4] Who needs another reason to optimize hormone levels?

IT'S A FACT

The US Preventive Services Task Force recommends mammograms every two years for women fifty to seventy-four years of age.

If you remember Becky from the start of chapter 10, her FSH number was around 150 IU/L when she first came to see me. That was an incredibly bad number for her body's health, especially her brain, and was causing her to age at warp speed. Like Becky, you want your FSH to be less than 23 IU/L. When your FSH number goes down, your LH will follow suit.

THE HORMONE HEALTH ZONE FOR ESTROGEN IN WOMEN

With all the known benefits of optimizing estradiol levels, from metabolism to weight loss to heart health to disease prevention, I'm amazed that most doctors stop all forms of estrogen therapy ten years after menopause. Perhaps this is because some people say that after taking this for long periods of time, the risks can outweigh the benefits, but I have not found that to be true with bioidentical estrogen. (And if doctors do prescribe estrogen, it usually is the pregnant horse hormone Premarin from pregnant mare urine, which your body cannot use correctly, thus causing many bad side effects.) That means millions of women around age sixty are suddenly and against their will experiencing warp-speed aging and brain degeneration. And it is all entirely unnecessary. The rapid aging and other negative symptoms don't have to happen. By optimizing hormone levels, women can usually stop the clock and, even better, turn back time!

IT'S A FACT

Interestingly women typically lose 30 percent of their skin collagen in the first five years after menopause. Estrogen reverses this trend and increases skin collagen, preventing wrinkles.[5]

For estrogen, there are several application options depending on your needs. Before I explain each application, I want to mention that in addition to taking estrogen, women (like men) need to take diindolylmethane (DIM), a natural supplement made from broccoli, to decrease estrone and help restore the 2-to-1 estradiol-to-estrone ratio. A 150 mg tablet once each day (twice a day for men) is sufficient. (See appendix F.)

Creams

Creams are quick, easy, and usually inexpensive. They usually require once-daily applications. For example, you can apply an estriol wrinkle cream once a day. Moisten your hands with water first, then apply 1 mL of cream to your face, your neck, and the backs of your hands. The estriol works wonders with collagen. And after a couple of months, there is often a huge difference! Some patients tell me their friends believed they had a face-lift. A compounding pharmacy makes it for my patients, and we call it wrinkle cream.

Creams usually require once-daily applications. However, as women age, their skin can lose some of its ability to absorb estrogen. So over time the dosage may need to increase or the application method may need to change.

Another cream is made to address vaginal dryness and atrophy. Women with this condition are miserable, but the estradiol cream works wonders in restoring the woman's vaginal fluids. Creams can be applied to the labia and vagina or may be applied to the skin. I usually recommend an estradiol/estriol cream in a 1-to-1 ratio (such as Biest) two or three times a week and for some, daily. Some women can only tolerate the estriol cream (they are less likely to start their periods again or have cramps, spotting, or breast tenderness, potential side effects of estradiol), which is the weakest estrogen, and is applied to the labia and vagina only once or twice a week.

Patches

Patches are also easy, fast, and usually inexpensive. They last for a few days, so you only need one or two per week, but some women say the patches come off after showering or swimming or they itch. It really depends on the person.

Sublingual tabs

Sublingual tabs are also quick, easy, and usually inexpensive. A tablet once a day under the tongue, or for better absorption between the lower lip and gum, dissolves in just minutes, making this an effective, easy, and problem-free method.

If you have not lowered your FSH level to less than 23 with optimal doses of the above, then shots or pellets are your next two options.

Shots

Once-a-week estradiol shots are quick and easy, usually not painful at all when using tiny needles, and also inexpensive.

Pellets

Pellets take a few minutes to insert under the skin, are virtually painless, and last for three to five months. It is the best delivery of estrogen (and testosterone) because it releases a consistent dosage. It is much pricier than the other methods, but it works incredibly well and usually brings down the FSH level faster and more consistently than any other method.

Again, the method of application is up to you. Talk with your doctor. Depending on the steps you need to take to optimize your estrogen levels, you can use one application method or another. Once you have chosen your preferred method of application, bioidentical hormones will do wonders in your body, usually bringing such dramatic change that women feel youthful and feminine again.

IT'S A FACT

Obesity increases estrone (the old lady estrogen) production.[6]

Whatever your age, it is never too late to start. But if I were to outline a proposed schedule for women, it would look something like this:

- At age forty, or perhaps sooner, optimize testosterone levels.
- At age forty-five start on progesterone.
- At age fifty (which is the average age for menopause) start on estrogen.

And you can keep this up until you are 100 or 120. Basically bioidentical hormone replacement therapy can keep you young and healthy for as long as you want.

WHEN ESTRADIOL IS RESTORED TO POWER

When your body is returned to its preferred ratio of 2-to-1 estradiol to estrone and FSH below 23 IU/L, your body usually comes alive! Many women say, "It is like someone turned the lights on again." What will that mean for you? All patients are different, but below are some common results my patients have experienced after reaching optimized estradiol levels.

For your metabolism:

- weight loss
- improved metabolism
- more energy and less fatigue
- improved muscle tone
- greater insulin sensitivity
- warmer body temperature
- prevention of obesity

For your heart:

- lower blood pressure
- improved blood flow
- protection from strokes
- bad (LDL) cholesterol lowered
- good (HDL) cholesterol raised
- protection from heart attack

For your skin:

- younger appearance
- fewer wrinkles
- fuller skin, including lips
- softer skin
- rehydration everywhere, including skin

For your brain:

- lower risk of Alzheimer's
- lower risk of Parkinson's
- lower risk of dementia
- increased neurotransmitters
- better memory
- greater focus
- ease of falling asleep and staying asleep
- improved sex drive
- better mood

For your bones:

- stronger bones
- protection from osteoporosis
- stronger teeth

For your eyes:

- protection from vision loss
- less light sensitivity
- less-dry eyes

For your breasts:

- perkier breasts
- reduced risk of breast cancer when combined with testosterone

For your hair and nails:

- thicker hair
- stronger nails

Whatever your symptoms, you can expect to improve them with optimized hormone levels, but your body will respond in different ways than the next person. That is always the case.

One great example is Cassie. She had had a hysterectomy in her late twenties and was only ever prescribed Premarin. The side effects were horrible for ten full years! She suffered from extreme mood swings, was on antidepressants, couldn't sleep, had thin hair, hated her premature wrinkles, and gained forty pounds. She looked like a heavy chain smoker, but she had never smoked in her life.

IT'S A FACT

Never take estrogen by mouth. It can raise the blood pressure, cause gallstones, elevate liver enzymes, cause weight gain, and increase one's craving for carbohydrates and starches. Instead use a topical (cream), sublingual tab (under the tongue), patch (on skin), shot (in thigh or buttock), or pellet (under the skin); just do not take a pill.[7]

Within two days of starting her bioidentical hormone therapy, which included testosterone, estradiol, and progesterone (to sleep), she said she felt like a different woman. She began to feel good and positive again, which was a shock to her system after ten years of feeling sad and miserable. Her wrinkles lessened significantly as her skin's collagen was partially restored. Her hair became thick and beautiful again, her belly fat disappeared, and her feminine curves returned. And she threw out her antidepressants. Her husband said it was a complete miracle.

I truly believe that when you get your FSH level to less than 23, you will have your own story to tell! I recommend that all women have a normal mammogram before starting estrogen replacement therapy (and have your mammogram repeated every one to two years), and all women should be on micronized progesterone unless they have had a hysterectomy.

IT'S A FACT

DIM increases the phase 1 detoxification of estrogens to 2-hydroxyestrone (2OHE1). The 2OH pathway has the lowest risk for breast cancer and does not stimulate cell growth. When 2OHE1 is then methylated in phase 2 detoxification in the liver, it is cancer protective. The dose of DIM needed to achieve this protective effect is 200–300 mg a day.

CHAPTER 13

EVEN MEN NEED SOME ESTROGEN

Unlike Joe from chapter 7, Richard did not elevate his estrogen levels by injecting high doses of testosterone into his body in an effort to create massive muscles. (Excessive testosterone aromatizes, or converts, to estradiol.) Richard did it naturally. He let gravity do all the hard work.

In high school Richard was a sports jock. He played in several sports, including soccer and track. In college he played Frisbee football and pickup basketball games every weekend. He was lean and mean, without an ounce of fat anywhere.

However, once he landed a job in the corporate world, he let go of the physical fitness side of things. When his thirty-inch waist hit forty inches, he bought a membership to a local gym, but his busy schedule kept his gym visits to a minimum. His waistline kept growing. At age forty-five Richard couldn't believe what had happened to him.

Firmly in the obese category, Richard came to see me, not because he wanted to lose weight but because he had read about obese men and he knew the statistics about diseases that followed obesity. He also had read about hormone replacement therapy, and he wanted to get started right away. He had already sold himself on what he needed.

"I'm guessing my testosterone levels are low," he began when we first met.

"And your estrogen levels are too high," I added.

The blood work from his prior doctor's charts was incomplete, so we ordered more to get a better picture of his overall health. Sure enough, his testosterone level was low, and his estradiol level was high. He clocked in at an estradiol level of 125 pg/mL. It should have been down to 20–70 pg/mL. I usually recommend a 20–50 pg/mL range. His total testosterone was 295 ng/dL. That was low! It should

161

have been at least 500 ng/dL. Optimized, it will be around 900–1100 ng/dL—which is the range Richard was probably at when he was in college—but can be as high as 1200.

"Your weight has you in an unfortunate position," I explained.

"Oh, I know," he stated. "And it's only going to get worse. My testosterone levels will get lower and lower, my estrogen levels will get higher, and most men like me end up with diseases such as type 2 diabetes, heart disease, prostate cancer, and more. I'm only thirty-six!"

Before I could say anything more, he added, "I've read a lot of articles about bioidentical hormone replacement therapy. I want to start now. What do I need to do?"

IT'S A FACT

Estrogen in men is made in the liver, muscle, brain, and fat cells. Obesity lowers testosterone levels and raises estrogen levels automatically and continuously.

"Overall good health definitely includes optimizing your hormone levels, but it's more than just hormones," I pointed out. "A healthy diet and exercise regimen is also a necessary part of the plan."

"Whatever I need to do, I'll do it," he said.

Thankfully Richard was only forty-five. If he were fifty-five, sixty-five, or seventy-five, the diseases he was trying to avoid would have probably already become a reality. He was right to take action when he did.

Still, I told him the best plan is to go slow. He needed a good dose of testosterone but was squeamish about shots and felt he couldn't remember to apply a testosterone cream or gel during his daily work schedule. The best option, he felt, was pellets.

IT'S A FACT

People who eat a lot of soy tend to have elevated estrogen levels and lowered testosterone levels. If you are trying to boost your testosterone levels, avoid soy.

He also went on the Keto Zone diet (see appendix F), as he really needed to cut down on his carbs and boost his proteins and healthy-fat intake. An exercise program of free weights and running short bursts on a treadmill at home were his preferred options. He also took the stairs instead of the elevator and went for a walk at lunchtime.

Within a few short weeks the change was beginning to take place. He noticed the muscle definition first in his arms and shoulders, but soon after, he saw it in his legs. His waist took the most work because of the belly fat that had accumulated, but he had lost almost thirty-five pounds before his second round of pellets. When he came in for new pellets at his six-month appointment, he looked completely different. He was almost unrecognizable in his new thirty-four-inch-waist business suit.

Now Richard only comes in twice a year. His testosterone levels stay right around 900 ng/dL, and his estrogen is down around 45 pg/mL. He takes 150 mg of diindolylmethane (DIM) twice a day to keep his estrogen conversion low and balanced. In all, he lost close to eighty pounds. And on his lunch walks, when he passes the basketball courts at the park, he looks like a sport jock who stepped into a business suit. He likes that.

ESTROGEN IS BOTH GOOD AND BAD FOR MEN

Estrogen is one of those things that is good for you in the proper amounts but bad for you if you have too much or too little of it. Just the right amount of estradiol is good for bone strength, sperm count, cholesterol metabolism, healthy libido, and clear thinking in the brain, just to name a few of the known values for estrogen in men.

Usually, however, it is too much estrogen in men that is much more common. This occurs when testosterone levels decrease due to aging, obesity, lifestyle, a lack of exercise, stress, endocrine disruptors, and so on. Too much estrogen has been found to promote abnormal clot formation or blood clots.[1] And excessive estrogen levels may also increase the risk of stroke.[2]

As testosterone lowers, estrogen usually rises. A healthy man usually needs to maintain at least a 10-to-1 ratio of testosterone (ng/dL) to estrogen (pg/mL). Richard and his total testosterone number of 295 ng/dL to estradiol number of 125 pg/mL meant his ratio was just over 2 to 1! That is extremely low and, as he understood, very bad for his health.

When his numbers were optimized to around 900 ng/dL (total testosterone) and 45 pg/mL (estradiol), his ratio was 20 to 1. And that's what he probably enjoyed when he was in his twenties. As Richard improved his lifestyle, principally his diet and exercise, his testosterone levels increased. Basically his body became more fit, and the testosterone pellets had a greater effect. Should he lower his dosage or maintain? He chose to maintain his dosage, as he loved the new "him" at his optimized levels.

When the ratio is far below 10 to 1, estrogen levels are too high, and that brings with it a host of ailments. Here are some of the symptoms I have seen in men who have too much estrogen in their bodies:

- brain fog
- lack of sex drive
- lack of erections
- low sperm count
- blood clots
- water retention
- gynecomastia (man boobs)

SIDE EFFECTS

There really are no negative side effects from bringing estrogen levels in men to the recommended "in range" level. Your health directly improves as a result.

There is also a higher risk for prostate cancer[3] and heart disease[4] when estrogen (estradiol) levels in men are too high.

Too little estrogen, and you also have a lack of sexual interest, few erections, and no libido. It is also not healthy for the brain to have super low estrogen levels, nor is brain fog a symptom that anyone enjoys.

Low estrogen levels do not only occur naturally. Sometimes they are the result of patients taking an aromatase inhibitor for too long without a doctor checking their estrogen numbers. Aromatase inhibitors are good because they lower estrogen numbers and decrease the testosterone-to-estrogen conversion, but without careful monitoring, estrogen levels can go too low. That is the beauty of DIM—it still lowers estrogen levels but will not push them too low.

I had one patient whose estradiol number was a mere 5 pg/mL. That was way too low. We took him off his aromatase inhibitor and put him on DIM while maintaining the testosterone therapy, and his estrogen levels increased and stayed in range.

The Hormone Health Zone for Estrogen in Men

Optimizing estrogen levels in men usually coincides with their testosterone levels. They are linked; raise testosterone, and estrogen usually rises; lower testosterone, and estrogen usually lowers. The goal is for at least a 10-to-1 ratio of testosterone (ng/dL) to estrogen (pg/mL).

When men start using testosterone cream, shots, or pellets, some of the testosterone aromatizes, or converts, to estrogen. Some men have excessive aromatization, especially older men and men who are obese. Remember, the normal range for estrogen (estradiol) in men is 20–70 pg/mL. When optimizing estradiol numbers in men, I recommend aiming for estradiol levels of 20–50 pg/mL. To stay in the estradiol hormone health zone, men will need to take DIM (150 mg twice a day). It is the safest way to lower estrogen without the fear of going too low.

For men who have never had their estrogen levels checked and believe they might have the symptoms of low or high estrogen, ask for blood work that gives you your estradiol level. Then you and your doctor will know what to do to treat it. Estrogen levels are usually pretty easy to treat in men.

It may be surprising that men need to watch their estrogen levels, but it's one of those things that you must be aware of. When we were learning to drive, we were all taught to watch for the "blind spots." Those spots aren't dangerous in and of themselves. But when you need to take action, the blind spots are suddenly very important.

Estrogen is a small player, but it can make a big impact if it's out of the normal range. Now you know more than enough to keep it in check!

CHAPTER 14

TESTOSTERONE ANSWERS FOR MEN

BIOLOGICALLY SPEAKING, TESTOSTERONE is what makes a man a man. It is made mainly in the testes but also in the adrenal glands. Most importantly, testosterone helps increase muscle mass and strength and helps burn fat. It also protects the brain, helps improve the memory, helps prevent and reverse depression and irritability, decreases inflammation throughout the body, increases energy, prevents feebleness and frailty, and helps maintain a good sex drive and strong, healthy erections.

PATIENT STORIES

Every man who optimizes his hormone levels has his own story, but here are four of my patients' stories to inspire you:

Lou's chronic pain

Lou was a house painter, and one day he fell off a roof and fractured his back. To say he lived in horrible chronic pain would be putting it mildly. He was in his mid-fifties when we optimized his hormones and put him on an anti-inflammation diet and a few anti-inflammatory supplements. After a few months his pain had reduced to what he described as "mild." He could get on with his life and resume his business, thanks in part to getting his testosterone levels back to what they were when he was twenty or twenty-five years old.

Jerry's sarcopenia

Jerry was eighty-two years old and shuffled everywhere he went. His rib cage was resting on his pelvis, and his belly was protuberant. He was almost frozen in that position, which made him look even older than he was. When we checked his testosterone level, it was in single digits at 9.0! Men need testosterone, and he had almost none in his system. It was hard to believe.

He began testosterone replacement therapy and a light exercise regimen of stretching and muscle building. Of course, prevention years
earlier would have been far better for Jerry, but even at his age it was
a huge improvement. His poor balance went away as his muscles
regained strength. He is still hunched over a bit, but he is spry and
athletic, and his belly is less protuberant, even in his condition. It also
made him look at least ten years younger, not to mention extending
his independence for who knows how many more years.

TESTOSTERONE-KILLING DRUGS FOR MEN

1. Cholesterol-lowering statin drugs
2. Certain BP-lowering drugs, including Aldactone, beta-
   blockers, and diuretics
3. Antidepressants, especially SSRIs

Walter's depression

Statistically more women battle depression than men, but Walter
was always down. He just turned sixty, was a small-business owner,
and worked incredibly hard, but he seemed permanently depressed.
Over the years, he had picked up prescriptions for two different antidepressants, high blood pressure medications, and a high cholesterol
medication. He was physically fit and in fact looked quite good, considering his age and health conditions. I checked his testosterone
levels, and sure enough, he was at the low end of normal. He tried
testosterone shots for a while but then opted for testosterone pellets.

When his testosterone hormone levels were optimized, everything
changed. His depression lifted completely, and he was able to stop
taking his antidepressants. They were his mainstay for years, but now
he no longer needed them. That was quite a change for him. Also, his
blood pressure and cholesterol improved, and he was able to reduce
his dosage of blood pressure medication and got off cholesterol medication as well. Also, his mood improved, his confidence returned, and
his business prospered.

Walter became high on life. In fact, he was in what he described as
a horrible marriage, but he didn't care. He felt so good and so excited

about living that he was not fazed by anything. He had found testosterone to be what it is: one of the best antidepressants in the world!

Bert's Parkinson's

Bert was seventy-five years old, and he suffered from severe Parkinson's. For ten years he dealt with increasing tremors and muscle loss and was frail and feeble. When we optimized his hormone levels simply by inserting testosterone pellets, the tremors subsided considerably. His muscle tone is back, he looks better every time he comes in for a checkup, and he is no longer feeble. Not only is this helping him cope with his Parkinson's; it is also helping protect his brain from more neuro-degeneration.

IT'S A FACT

When people use certain drugs or smoke, these chemicals boost dopamine levels in the brain and are highly addictive. Testosterone in the body has a similar dopamine effect in the brain. When testosterone levels are optimized, you feel really good, and that helps tremendously with depression for both men and women.

Every doctor who uses bioidentical hormone replacement therapy has stories about how patients suddenly went from a diseased state to a state of health in one area or another. Some of the stories are hard to believe because the health improvements are so dramatic, but that is the power of hormones at work in our bodies.

This is especially true of testosterone. It is the hormone with the most health benefits mentally, emotionally, and physically. It boosts energy and decreases inflammation and chronic pain. Without sufficient testosterone, our bodies pay an incredible price.

I call it the "home run hormone" because when the testosterone level is optimized in men, it's like flipping on all the key breaker switches (figuratively speaking) in the body as the body usually starts to heal when combined with an anti-inflammatory or Keto Zone diet. (See appendix F.)

Symptoms of Low Testosterone in Men

Although there are some similarities, the symptoms of low and suboptimal testosterone in men are slightly different than in women. They include:

- brain fog
- weight gain
- lack of focus
- less drive
- indecisiveness
- need for afternoon naps
- cloud of depression that does not lift
- irritability and grumpiness
- decreased ability to have an orgasm
- diminished job performance
- increased sleepiness after dinner
- less strength, stamina, and endurance
- loss of competitiveness
- belly fat and love handles
- insomnia
- desire to make the couch the new hangout (couch potato)
- fatigue
- decreased sex drive
- loss of morning erections
- aching muscles and joints
- muscle turning to fat
- loss of confidence
- rise in bad cholesterol
- less enjoyment in life
- increased risk of heart disease
- sarcopenia (muscle loss)
- prediabetes and type 2 diabetes

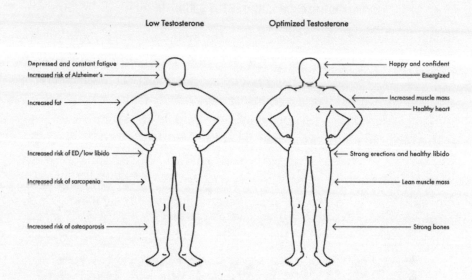

Low Testosterone · Optimized Testosterone

Depressed and constant fatigue → · ← Happy and confident
Increased risk of Alzheimer's → · ← Energized
Increased fat → · ← Increased muscle mass
· ← Healthy heart
Increased risk of ED/low libido → · ← Strong erections and healthy libido
Increased risk of sarcopenia → · ← Lean muscle mass
Increased risk of osteoporosis → · ← Strong bones

Nobody wants any of these symptoms. Unfortunately from age thirty-five onward men lose 1 percent of their testosterone production per year.[1] Some say it's as much as 5 percent. If we go with 1 percent, that still breaks down to a testosterone loss of about 10 percent per decade. So even if it's 1 percent each year, that is way too much! Men need their testosterone.

Based on this gradual annual testosterone loss, most men will start seeing some side effects of low testosterone around age fifty. Add in obesity, prediabetes, type 2 diabetes, nutritional deficiencies, chronic stress, medications, diseases, diet, increased exposure to endocrine disruptors, and a lack of exercise, and the rate of testosterone loss speeds up exponentially.

PREVENTION AND CURE

Men need to be fully aware of what is happening in their bodies as they age, like Richard from chapter 13, who read about hormone replacement therapy. The old Benjamin Franklin axiom "An ounce of prevention is worth a pound of cure" could not be more aptly spoken than when it comes to testosterone. And since millions of men in the United States—half of all men over the age of fifty—may suffer from low testosterone, that makes it something men cannot and should not ignore.[2] Consider these facts:

Testosterone fact 1—It helps keep your body lean and muscular.

With testosterone-deficient men testosterone usually makes a pretty big impact. In one study testosterone replacement therapy helped healthy older men with low or suboptimal testosterone raise their lean body mass and lower their fat mass. What is more, testosterone improved overall body strength, performance, sexual function, and mood.[3] The fatter men get, the lower their testosterone levels usually go, and the higher their estrogen usually goes, which makes them fatter still, causing even lower testosterone levels, and their health deteriorates further.[4]

THE TESTOSTERONE/ CHOLESTEROL LINK

Testosterone is made from cholesterol in your body. I have found from over thirty-four years' experience practicing medicine that if you lower your cholesterol with a statin drug, you also usually lower your testosterone.

Testosterone fact 2—It helps strengthen your bones.

Testosterone keeps bones dense and slows down the bone loss that typically comes with age.[5] That lines up with what I've seen in my practice because men who suffer from bone loss and/or osteoporosis usually also have low testosterone.[6]

IT'S A FACT

Alcohol consumption can increase estradiol levels in men. Elevated estradiol lowers libido, converts testosterone to estrogen, and grows man boobs. Avoid alcohol, or drink small amounts, and not daily.

Testosterone fact 3—It helps protect you from dementia and Alzheimer's disease.

Maintaining a healthy level of testosterone reduces the risk of dementia. It may actually prevent Alzheimer's.[7] Testosterone is a vital ingredient for effective brain chemistry.[8]

Testosterone fact 4—It helps protect you against prostate cancer.

The myth that high levels of testosterone cause prostate cancer came from a single study back in 1941,[9] which was admittedly flawed. For decades since then the myth has lived on, and it is often still claimed that low testosterone levels will protect you from prostate cancer, but that is not the truth. Instead, they actually increase the risk. Testosterone treatment does not increase the risk of prostate cancer, even with men who are already at risk.[10] The fact is, prostate cancer is more common with low testosterone levels, and those low testosterone levels are found to actually increase the severity of cancer.[11] To refute the long-held belief that testosterone increases the risk of prostate cancer, a collaboration of eighteen studies showed no connection between increased risk of prostate cancer and higher testosterone levels.[12] In sum, men can put the fear and worry that high testosterone levels cause prostate cancer to rest.[13]

Testosterone fact 5—It helps you maintain sexual function.

For men and women, maintaining sexual function as we age is necessary. Sufficient levels of testosterone are a required part of that.[14]

Testosterone fact 6—It helps your heart stay healthy.

Heart disease is still the number one killer of men and women. When hormone levels are optimized, especially testosterone levels, weight usually goes down, and energy levels go up, which are both required for good heart health. Cholesterol levels usually also improve. When testosterone levels are optimized, the risk of heart disease and death are drastically reduced.[15] Also, one interesting fact about the heart is that there are more testosterone receptors on cardiac muscle than any other muscle in the body. In other words, the heart needs testosterone more than any other muscle in the body, especially since it is always beating and never really rests. Testosterone also increases nitric oxide, which supports healthy blood flow and healthy blood pressure.

Testosterone fact 7—It is great for overall disease protection and prevention.

One recent study found that men treated with testosterone had a measurable 24 percent decrease in heart attacks, a 36 percent decrease in strokes, and an amazing 56 percent lower risk of dying from other causes, including cancer.[16] And another study of thirty thousand middle-aged and older men found that testosterone therapy did not increase the risk of blood clots.[17]

Testosterone fact 8—It prevents and treats depression.

Testosterone both prevents and treats depression in many men mainly by boosting dopamine levels. There are many studies demonstrating that testosterone improves mood and reduces depression significantly.

TOP TWELVE REASONS MEN WANT TO OPTIMIZE TESTOSTERONE LEVELS

I've just covered some of the many facts that surround testosterone. But what about real people? What do real patients care about? Here are the top twelve reasons my male patients have said they want to optimize their testosterone levels. (I find the women who love them wholeheartedly agree.)

1. **"I want my muscles back."** Muscle that was lost can be rebuilt, and once-toned bodies can be fit again. This is the best way to stay young.

2. **"I have to stop this fatigue cycle."** Greater stamina, energy, endurance, and strength can be regained with higher testosterone levels. Being a couch potato is not the life anyone wants!

3. **"I gotta lose weight."** Gaining weight, especially in the belly area, is a common sign of low testosterone. Boosting testosterone helps turn up the metabolism and burn off the fat. Type 2 diabetics usually have low

testosterone, but optimized testosterone levels (along with diet and exercise) help overcome type 2 diabetes.

4. **"I need to lower my cholesterol level."** Testosterone helps lower the bad cholesterol and raise the good cholesterol.

5. **"I simply must get my manhood back."** Many men suffer from erectile dysfunction (ED), often due to low testosterone. Raise testosterone levels, and ED is usually improved and sometimes gone.

6. **"I'm sick of constant brain fog."** When testosterone levels are optimized, the brain fog usually lifts. This also brings increased focus, sharper clarity, and improved decision making.

7. **"I need to beat depression."** Usually the best remedy for depression is to boost testosterone levels. As depression lifts, typically irritability and grumpiness go along with it.

8. **"I can't sleep, and I really need to sleep!"** Insomnia has many causes, but low testosterone allows cortisol levels to rise, and that usually decreases your ability to sleep at night. Optimizing testosterone usually improves sleep and helps lower nighttime cortisol levels.

9. **"I know I need to protect my brain."** There are many memory-related illnesses, including dementia and Alzheimer's, that are positively impacted by optimized testosterone levels.

10. **"I need help with my arthritis."** The anti-inflammatory effects of optimized testosterone levels bring great relief to many arthritis sufferers as well as patients with chronic pain.

11. **"I need to reset my adrenals."** When adrenal glands are stressed and overworked, optimizing testosterone levels will usually help give the adrenal glands the rest they need so they can heal. It helps to reset the adrenal glands.

12. **"I want to stay out of a nursing home."** Optimized
    levels of testosterone prevent and reverse bone and
    muscle loss (osteoporosis and sarcopenia), two of the
    primary reasons why people end up in nursing homes.
    It also protects the brain from dementia, and nursing
    homes are full of patients with dementia.

And there you have it. What is your reason for wanting to optimize
your testosterone levels?

THE HORMONE HEALTH ZONE FOR TESTOSTERONE IN MEN

Numerous diseases and countless symptoms are positively impacted
when testosterone levels are optimized. If you are battling some of
the symptoms and diseases associated with low or suboptimal testosterone, then it is time to boost your testosterone levels up to what they
were when you were in your twenties.

What will happen? Most likely a lot of improvement in your health,
energy, and enjoyment in life will happen! The hormone health zone
is where symptoms and diseases often lessen or disappear entirely. It
is also the place where many people get their lives back! Men, you
want to know your total testosterone and free testosterone numbers.
Here are the normal ranges for both:

Total testosterone ranges in men

According to LabCorp, its recommended range for men (over age
eighteen) for total testosterone is 264–916 ng/dL. A few years ago it
was 348–1197, but LabCorp recently lowered it. Another lab, Quest
Diagnostics, has a similar range for total testosterone: 250–1100 ng/dL.
When men optimize their total testosterone (pushed to the upper
range of normal) to the levels they were at when they were in their
twenties, total testosterone numbers will be closer to 500–1100 ng/dL.

Any man "in range" with a total testosterone number that is low
or suboptimal (250–500 ng/dL) is most likely going to have negative
symptoms or is developing those symptoms. A man's body needs more
testosterone than the lower end of these ranges can afford. Remember,
the symptoms mean more than the range does, so if you have some of
the symptoms of low testosterone in your body, there is a reason for it.

Some men need their testosterone optimized even higher, to 750–1100, even 1200, to eliminate most or all of their low testosterone symptoms.

Free testosterone ranges in men

The same lab companies recommend these ranges for free testosterone in men:

LabCorp:

- age twenty to twenty-nine: 9.3–26.5 pg/mL
- age thirty to thirty-nine: 8.7–25.1 pg/mL
- age forty to forty-nine: 6.8–21.5 pg/mL
- age fifty to fifty-nine: 7.2–24.0 pg/mL
- over age fifty-nine: 6.6–18.1 pg/mL

Quest Diagnostics:

- age eighteen to sixty-nine: 46–224 pg/mL
- age seventy to eighty-nine: 6–73 pg/mL

Optimized free testosterone levels will look more like this:

- free testosterone for men: 150–224 pg/mL

The concentration of free testosterone is usually very low and usually less than 2 percent of the total testosterone concentration. Remember, the free testosterone is the active testosterone. Approximately sixty percent of total testosterone is bound to SHBG, and once bound, it cannot be released and used inside cells. About 38 percent of testosterone is bound to albumin[18] and can become free testosterone again if supplemented with adequate DIM, usually 150 mg twice a day.

Again, most men at the low-to-suboptimal range are going to really be hurting. But when free testosterone and total testosterone are optimized, that is where amazing results take place. For example, when it comes to protection from heart disease, it was found that cardiovascular risks dropped dramatically when total testosterone levels were optimized above 550 ng/dL.[19]

IT'S A FACT

Men are less likely than women to get osteoporosis, Hashimoto's, or dementia. Men have eight to ten times more testosterone in their bodies than women and produce twenty times more testosterone than women do.[20] Therefore, it stands to reason that a key preventive for these diseases is testosterone.

When you were twenty-five years of age, it's unlikely that you worried about your cholesterol levels, heart disease, depression, sexual function, memory-related illnesses, muscle degeneration, or even your weight. You were too busy living and enjoying life! Optimizing your hormone levels, especially testosterone, can potentially bring back much of the same zest for living, health, disease prevention, strength, and hope that you once enjoyed.

TESTS AND TREATMENT PLANS

When men reach a point where they can no longer ignore their symptoms (we men are masters at ignoring symptoms until they become obvious to all), then and only then will they go to a doctor. Hopefully that doctor is one who practices bioidentical hormone replacement therapy.

If you are having trouble finding a doctor who practices bioidentical hormone replacement therapy, you can find doctors online. There are several websites listed in appendix F to assist you in finding a doctor who is knowledgeable in bioidentical hormones.

Begin with the right tests. Many doctors, even those who do not practice hormone replacement therapy, will help you get the hormonal lab tests that you need. The right lab tests will most likely pinpoint the issue behind your symptoms. Low testosterone levels, both free and total, are the primary causes of so many symptoms that it is safe to say, "I'm experiencing many of the symptoms of low testosterone." (Of course, your doctor will want to run the tests to find out!) And if either total or free testosterone is low, usually the other is low as well.

In total, I recommend the following hormone tests:

- total testosterone
- free testosterone
- TSH
- TPO antibodies
- rT3

- SHBG
- estradiol
- PSA
- free T3 level

I also check a complete blood count, a comprehensive metabolic panel, a lipid panel, a hemoglobin A1C, a 25OHD3 (vitamin D_3) level, a CRP, a B_{12} level, and a urinalysis.

Men have several different options for testosterone replacement therapy.

Sublingual tabs

There is no natural testosterone that you can take by mouth as a pill except sublingual testosterone tabs that are compounded at a compounding pharmacy. Sublingual tabs are taken by placing one tab under the tongue, or even better between the lower lip and gum, two to three times per day. Taking testosterone orally (not sublingually) usually elevates liver enzymes and may cause a drug-induced hepatitis. That's why I recommend the creams, gels, shots, and pellets as the preferred ways to administer testosterone.

Creams and gels

Transdermal creams and gels are the most common form of testosterone therapy. The dosage is usually 50–200 pg of testosterone in 0.5–1 mL of cream applied to the skin behind the knee or shoulder once a day. The best place to apply it is the back of the knee, where it is hairless, and rotating sides, or the shoulder. If men can get their testosterone levels up with a cream, they will often do it, as it's painless. Shots and pellets raise testosterone levels very well but are often pricier than other methods and more painful. Some men hate injections and minor surgical procedures such as pellets. Testosterone creams are able to provide better absorption through the skin than gels. Creams also provide moisturizers to the skin and do not dry out the skin like alcohol-based gels. (Creams and gels of testosterone can be accidentally transferred to children and women, causing masculinizing effects.) Creams may also raise dihydrotestosterone (DHT) levels more than injections and pellets. DHT can trigger male pattern baldness, prostate enlargement, and acne. Creams and gels can also increase estrogen levels. Though shots and pellets are usually the main way to boost testosterone levels up into the optimal range, the new cream base (Atrevis base) delivers testosterone through the skin by using several naturally derived permeation enhancers. It is nice to be able to now optimize testosterone levels without shots or pellets, as some patients do not like the shots or pellets.

IT'S A FACT

AndroGel is the most prescribed testosterone in the world but is quite expensive. A much less expensive option is testosterone transdermal cream, especially in the new Atrevis base found at compounding pharmacies.

Shots

More and more, injections are becoming less painful and easier to give. They last for several days, so just one or two shots a week are usually sufficient. These shots can now be given subcutaneously with very small needles and are injected into the lateral thigh, buttock, or deltoid muscle. They are usually almost painless and rarely associated with bruising. Some compounding pharmacies will preload the syringes for you so no measuring is required. Either way, shots are a very effective method when it comes to optimizing testosterone levels.

TESTOSTERONE CLINICS

Typically just men go to testosterone clinics, and the usual method of testosterone application is shots (once or twice per week). The clinics meet a need, but they are usually only optimizing (sometimes pushing beyond optimized) one hormone: testosterone. Optimizing all hormones and diet, nutrition, a healthy lifestyle, and so on, are not part of the service, nor do they meet other challenges, such as DHT, hair loss, increased estrogen levels, and more. If you

do use a testosterone clinic, make sure you are optimizing
all your other hormones as well.

Pellets

Though often much pricier that the other methods, pellets by far are
the easiest way to boost your testosterone levels. Five to ten 200 mg
pellets every six months, and you don't have to think about it again. A
pellet is about the size of a grain of rice, and it is inserted in the hip
area and is based on your body weight and testosterone level. It is a
minor surgical procedure, but it is fast, easy, and usually painless.

Other Factors That Affect Testosterone Therapy

In addition to testing the hormones you want to optimize, always
remember to keep an eye on the other factors that can adversely affect
the testosterone therapy. For men that includes:

Estradiol

Men on testosterone therapy may also be elevating their estradiol
levels. (See chapter 13 for more details.) Keeping the estradiol level
between 20 and 50 pg/mL is ideal.[21]

SHBG

Approximately 60 percent of testosterone is bound to SHBG in
healthy young men.[22] When testosterone is bound to SHBG, it can
no longer be used by the body. Elderly men usually have much higher
SHBG levels and decreased levels of free testosterone, which is the
testosterone that can be used by the body. Men, if your SHBG is high,
you will probably need a higher dose of testosterone to optimize your
free testosterone, or else you could have a high normal testosterone
level and still have numerous symptoms of low testosterone because
the majority of your testosterone is bound by SHBG. For men with
low testosterone symptoms and high normal total testosterone levels,
be sure to check your SHBG and free testosterone levels.

DHT

Testosterone is converted to DHT—which I call "testosterone's
nasty little cousin"—by the enzyme 5-alpha-reductase. DHT is very
masculinizing and causes your voice to lower at puberty and is

responsible for hair growth in your groin, face, and chest. It's also the main cause of male pattern baldness, enlargement of the prostate, and acne. Keeping an eye on testosterone's nasty little cousin, DHT, is recommended if you are developing these symptoms. It can usually be controlled by putting testosterone cream on a hairless area (such as behind the knee), decreasing the dose of testosterone, changing to pellets, or using herbs or meds to minimize conversion.

DIM

For lowering estradiol, taking diindolylmethane (DIM), a natural supplement made from broccoli, will help lower estradiol levels that may try to creep up. This is especially true for men as they age.[23] Taking 150–200 mg of DIM twice a day is usually sufficient to keep estradiol levels in check. Some men may need to take it three times a day, and very rarely some men need a low dose of Arimidex, which is another estrogen blocker, or aromatase inhibitor. (See appendix F.)

TESTOSTERONE LEVELS ARE DROPPING

At this point you might be thinking, "How do I know if I need testosterone replacement therapy?"

IT'S A FACT

Basically, despite all the myths, fears, and faulty studies, bioidentical optimized testosterone levels will usually not cause hair growth, hair loss, aggression, acne, gynecomastia (man boobs), sleep apnea, cancer, stroke, or heart attacks. Rather, it is high-dose synthetic, anabolic testosterone abuse that is associated with these adverse side effects.[24]

That is a valid question. The answer is going to be based on your symptoms and your needs, but if you are looking for a number, you can call 500 ng/dL your cutoff point. If your total testosterone number is less than 500 ng/dL and you are beginning to notice some symptoms of low testosterone, you have your answer. At that point I would suggest that you start testosterone replacement therapy.

This applies whether you are thirty-nine or ninety-nine years old.

You do not need to go through life or finish out your life battling the countless symptoms of low testosterone. Everyone else might, but you don't have to! Across the board, testosterone levels are dropping in American men[25] and have been for decades.

And if that isn't enough, look at the increased incidence of heart disease, obesity, type 2 diabetes, sarcopenia, osteoporosis, dementia, Parkinson's, and Alzheimer's. These and many other diseases are increasing *exactly* in sync with the decline of our testosterone levels!

As we have discussed throughout this book, there are many reasons why our testosterone levels are tanking. For most, it is a combination of being overweight, nutritional deficiencies, chronic stress, medications, diseases, diet, hormone disruptors, and age. Odds are, your testosterone levels are not what they should be.

SIDE EFFECTS

- **What about the prostate?** I start patients with a PSA test. If it is over 2.5, I have them meet with a urologist to make sure they do not have early prostate cancer. (If they have prostate cancer, I do not give them testosterone replacement therapy.) And we monitor PSA on a regular basis. **The answer:** Protect the prostate with herbs and supplements.

- **What about atrophy (shrinking) of the testicle?** Some men get atrophy of the testicle with testosterone therapy. Pellets usually do not cause it, shots will, and creams may. **The answer:** HCG 200–500 units subcutaneously two or three times a week to maintain testicle size. It is a prescription, but doctors can prescribe it to prevent testicular atrophy.

- **What about baldness, acne, and prostate enlargement?** Cream or gel application, because it is applied to the skin, sometimes increases dihydrotestosterone (DHT), which may cause male pattern baldness, acne, and prostate enlargement. **The answer:** There are several supple-

ments (pumpkin seed oil, saw palmetto, beta sitosterol,
and more) and prescriptions that help block DHT.

If you are taking statin drugs to lower your cholesterol (at your doctor's recommendation no doubt), there is usually no chance that your
testosterone levels are healthy! As I mentioned earlier, testosterone is
made from cholesterol in your body, so if you decrease the cholesterol,
you usually decrease the testosterone as well. Thankfully, as you also
know, optimized testosterone levels will usually lower the bad cholesterol and raise the good cholesterol in your body.

If you are fighting obesity, the increased fat around the internal
organs increases the conversion of testosterone to estrogen.[26] That
means your body continues producing excessive estrogen, which will
further compound obesity and create a whole list of negative symptoms and diseases in your body. Diet, exercise, and testosterone
replacement therapy are vital to break this vicious cycle.

If you want to stay out of a nursing home, it's a good idea to keep
your testosterone levels optimized. Letting muscle turn to fat is one
of the surest ways to lose your independence. Keep your testosterone
levels up and exercise. I have some eighty-year-olds who can do a
three-minute plank! Most people can hardly do it for sixty seconds.
Maintain your muscle, and you maintain your overall health.

The testosterone-lowering trend is only going to continue, and there
is nothing we are doing as a society to stop it. The only defense is your
own defense, but you get to choose how you want to live your life.

CHAPTER 15

OPTIMIZING GROWTH HORMONE

MENTION GROWTH HORMONE, and people usually think of children and teens who are much shorter than their peers and who have a growth hormone deficiency and actually need growth hormone injections. But that is only part of the picture.

Susan and Nick, two separate patients from two different states, also thought the same thing and were surprised when I explained that human growth hormone (HGH) would help meet their health and longevity goals.

"I'm not getting any taller," Nick had said. "I'm only getting older. Why would I need growth hormone?"

Similarly, Susan had argued, "I'm seventy-eight, and my body is aging faster than the rest of me. I need to stay independent for as long as I can. I need to be fit and healthy to do that, and how would growth hormone help me achieve those goals?"

Nick was in his mid-sixties and pastored a growing church up north. Staying in shape meant more time to help people, impact their lives, and accomplish the things he believed God had for him to do.

Susan had lived alone since her husband died several years earlier, and she had no family nearby. She desperately wanted to stay active and to stay out of a nursing home. However, she had osteoporosis and knew if something didn't change, her days of independence were numbered.

Both had different goals, but both were highly motivated. Still, they both asked, "Why do I need growth hormones?" As for timing, only after we optimized all their other hormones did I test them for growth hormone deficiency.

WHAT GROWTH HORMONE DOES FOR YOU

The human growth hormone originates in the pituitary gland and secretes into our bodies about five times every day, which makes it a bit of a challenge to measure accurately. It stimulates growth in children and teens, peaking in intensity during the teen years. But that is not all it does. Usually at about eighteen years of age your epiphyseal plates fuse, and you will not grow taller, even with growth hormone. But the human growth hormone continues to work in your body as you age, performing the following tasks:

- repairs and thickens thin skin
- boosts metabolism
- burns off fat
- provides energy
- rejuvenates cells
- strengthens nails and hair
- grows muscle
- strengthens the immune system

- repairs damaged tissue
- makes bones dense and strong
- improves brain function
- boosts sexual performance
- improves memory
- helps heal wounds
- lowers cholesterol
- helps rejuvenate important organs

When people hear this list of benefits, they nod their heads in approval and, like both Susan and Nick, say wholeheartedly, "I certainly do want and need that for my body."

Our problem is that the production of growth hormone in our bodies quickly declines as we age. I have read numerous studies reporting that after twenty, thirty, or forty years of age our growth hormone levels drop by 50 percent every seven, ten, or twenty years. While there is disagreement on the actual age that the decline starts or how rapidly our growth hormone levels decline, there is no disagreement about the fact that we lose our growth hormone substantially as we age.

If we were to pick the middle ground and say that we lose 50 percent of our growth hormone every ten years from age thirty onward, that would mean Nick and Susan have about 10 percent and 5 percent, respectively, left in their systems. That is not enough. They need more than that if they hope to reach and maintain their health goals. And you need more than that yourself!

Testing and Boosting Your HGH Levels

As we age, common symptoms of low or suboptimal growth hormone levels begin to emerge, such as:

- saggy, baggy, thin skin
- weaker muscles and decreased strength
- lethargy and fatigue
- slower metabolism with weight gain
- increased degree and frequency of mood swings
- slow-healing wounds
- decreased energy and stamina
- memory loss
- frailty
- difficulty sleeping
- decreased libido
- anxiety and depression
- decreased sexual function
- difficulty concentrating

These symptoms do indeed look similar to many of the low or suboptimal testosterone symptoms. That is certainly the case, but how do you know if low testosterone, low growth hormone levels, or something else entirely is to blame for your symptoms?

There are two recognized tests you can take, screening tests, actually, to see if your growth hormone levels are low. One test is the glucagon stimulation test, and the other is an insulin tolerance test. Doctors are not supposed to prescribe growth hormone unless one or the other of these tests is abnormal.

Most likely, as there are very few adults who are actually deficient in growth hormone, your lab numbers will put you in the normal range of insulin-like growth factor 1 (IGF-1)—a screening test for growth hormone deficiency—which, according to Quest Diagnostics, will be around:

AGE	MALE	FEMALE
Fifty-one to sixty	87–225 ng/mL	92–190 ng/mL
Sixty-one to seventy	75–228 ng/mL	87–178 ng/mL
Seventy-one to eighty	31–187 ng/mL	25–171 ng/mL
Eighty-one to ninety	68–157 ng/mL	31–162 ng/mL

Again, you will probably be in range regardless of your age because the lab ranges are set so low. That usually does little to make your symptoms go away, nor does it help you attain your goals. Even if your IGF-1 levels are low, doctors are not supposed to prescribe growth hormone unless one of the two tests mentioned above (the glucagon stimulation test or the insulin tolerance test) shows low growth hormone levels, but that is extremely rare.

Since the clinical features of adult growth hormone deficiency are nonspecific, growth hormone stimulation testing is required in order for a physician to prescribe growth hormone. As I mentioned, the glucagon stimulation test and the insulin tolerance test are the two accepted tests in the United States for adult growth hormone deficiency. The insulin tolerance test (ITT) is the diagnostic test of choice, but it is not advised as a procedure for the elderly or for patients with ischemic heart disease or seizures. In other words, usually the very patients who need growth hormone can't take the test because the test is too dangerous for them. The test involves giving a good dose of insulin IV (0.1 units/kg) and then measuring the glucose, GH, and cortisol levels at baseline and every thirty minutes for three hours.

The glucagon stimulation test is the main alternative to the ITT. The vast majority of adults tested by these tests do not meet the criteria for adult growth hormone deficiency, even if their IGF-1 level is very low.

The IGF-1 test is an indirect way of measuring the amount of growth hormone produced in the body. Growth hormone is able to stimulate the production and release of IGF-1 as well as other insulin-like growth factors that stimulate growth in most cells in the body. IGF-1 levels peak in puberty and then decline in adulthood. IGF-1 levels, unlike growth hormone levels, are stable throughout the day. Growth hormone is transported in the blood, mainly by the IGF-binding proteins IGFBP-2 and IGFBP-3. These proteins help maintain higher IGF-1 levels in the blood and help minimize swings in the levels.

Nick had naturally low IGF-1 levels, but he was still "in range." Even Susan was still in range, though she was admittedly at the low end of the range. In both cases doctors would not prescribe either of them growth hormone.

Most likely, just like Nick and Susan, you will:

- not be growth hormone deficient or low in IGF-1
- not be below the established range for IGF-1

But that is not a problem. It would certainly seem like one, but here is something unique about our human growth hormone (HGH) itself. Our bodies seldom lose the ability to make enough growth hormone, but usually we lose the ability to release adequate amounts of growth hormone.

Your body can usually produce growth hormone, but as you age, you may lose the ability to release adequate amounts, and eventually IGF-1 levels become low or low normal. What our bodies lose as we age are the signals that tell the pituitary gland to release more growth hormone.

In essence, the voice crying, "Release more growth hormone!" goes silent. And since the pituitary gland never gets the call to release more, it assumes there is no need for more. This is one of those times when no news is not good news!

The answer is peptides. You usually need a prescription for these because they are usually injected subcutaneously and tell your pituitary gland to release more growth hormone into your body. (Peptides can also be in pill form—MK-677—if that is preferred.) These are usually prescribed by antiaging physicians.

Several effective peptides are:

- ipamorelin (mild and affordable)
- sermorelin (most common and very affordable)
- ibutamoren—MK-677 (ideal to combat sarcopenia, muscle loss, and bone loss, and is in oral form)

In addition to peptides, another way to send a message to the pituitary gland is with amino acid secretagogues, which can be found in most health food stores. Like their name, the amino acid secretagogues simply tell the pituitary gland to secrete more of something, in this case, more growth hormones. Several HGH-boosting secretagogues include:

- lysine/arginine
- arginine/ornithine
- glutamine

- GABA
- SeroVital

I have found that younger people under fifty usually do great with amino acid secretagogues and that older people, especially over age sixty, usually need a greater boost of growth hormone secretion, which peptides provide.

But with both peptides and amino acid secretagogues, the pituitary receives the message and usually starts pumping out more growth hormone. And as a result, you usually get what you want, and that is muscle growth, an increase in lean body mass, a loss of fat, better sleep, organ rejuvenation, a sharper brain, and much more.

MORE ABOUT HGH

HGH is a peptide hormone composed of 191 amino acids that is secreted by the anterior pituitary gland as well as regulated by the anterior pituitary. HGH stimulates IGF-1 when it binds to growth hormone receptors throughout the body, and that stimulates the growth of muscle and loss of fat.

Growth hormone secretagogues are peptides that induce the secretion of growth hormone. Most of these peptides should be injected subcutaneously at bedtime except for ibutamoren (MK-677), which is an oral peptide, again, taken at bedtime. There are two types of growth hormone peptide secretagogues:

- agonist of the growth hormone secretagogue receptor (GHSR), including ipamorelin, ibutamoren (MK-677), GHRP-2, GHRP-6

- agonist of growth hormone-releasing hormone receptor (GHRHR), including sermorelin, CJC-1295, and tesamorelin

Combining GHSR peptide, such as ipamorelin, with a GHRHR peptide, such as CJC-1295, will usually produce a greater release of GH and IGF-1. They have a synergistic effect that helps the body release its own stored-up growth hormone.

GETTING GREAT RESULTS

Growth hormone usually has an amazing effect with people who suffer from chronic or degenerative diseases, such as sarcopenia, osteoporosis, and fibromyalgia. The muscle and bone regeneration are particularly impactful.

With Susan, the peptide secretagogues (in addition to optimizing her other hormone levels, especially her testosterone) increased her growth hormone count considerably. Her bone degeneration stopped. Her diet and exercise program meshed well with her increase in energy levels, and before she knew it, her muscles were becoming firmer, and her weight declined. Her bones began to strengthen and get denser, and her skin tightened! That was exactly what she needed.

SIDE EFFECTS

Side effects of HGH are rare, but include:

- carpal tunnel syndrome
- fluid retention in hands and feet
- tingling and numbness of the skin
- muscle aches
- joint aches
- headaches

Nick had different goals. The peptides, along with optimizing his hormone levels, helped him think more clearly and made his brain even sharper. He also gained better muscle definition than he had ever had previously. In fact, his workout trainers noticed his muscle growth and overall body toning and wanted to know what he was doing to get such great results. He also reported much improved sleep and felt more refreshed.

Peptides really turn up the fat burning when combined with optimized levels of testosterone and thyroid. In addition to incredibly quick fat burning, my patients have experienced smoother skin, improved muscle tone, and fewer wrinkles. Combine peptides with a healthy lifestyle (diet, exercise, decreased stress, good sleep, and so on), and the results can be incredible. When you can stop and then reverse symptoms that once seemed impossible to fix, that is an amazing thing!

Of course, getting "great results" is attractive to anyone, especially bodybuilders who want to quickly build muscle and burn fat. In the eighties and nineties, taking large doses of growth hormones (not just peptides or secretagogues) along with steroids enabled bodybuilders to get incredibly large muscles. As you would also expect, negative side effects—such as edema, carpal tunnel, joint swelling, water retention, increased incidences for type 2 diabetes, and even cancer—followed the excessive doses of growth hormones.

This is a case of taking too much of something good. It damaged their bodies, but it also gave human growth hormones (HGH) a bad name. If people call HGH "one of those bodybuilder things," you know why, but that does not negate the fact that virtually all of us eventually need more growth hormone in our bodies as we age. Since then a lot of research has been done to show just how beneficial growth hormone is when used properly. Here are some examples.

HGH benefit 1: lean body, less fat

For both men and women, multiple studies have found that increasing growth hormone levels can not only restore but also increase overall muscle mass. One study of sixteen women, whose ages ranged from seventy to seventy-three, found that only four weeks of increased growth hormone levels from HGH supplementation improved overall lean body mass and simultaneously caused a significant decrease in body fat.[1]

HGH benefit 2: more muscle, stronger bones

In another study twenty-one healthy men whose ages ranged from sixty-one to eighty-one increased growth hormone levels with HGH supplementation over a six-month period. The results were astounding: an 8.8 percent increase in lean body mass, a 14.4 percent reduction in adipose tissue mass, and a 1.6 percent increase in average lumbar spine vertebral bone density. The researchers concluded: "The increase in adipose-tissue mass and the thinning of the skin that occur in older men are caused in part by reduced activity of the [human] growth hormone-IGF-1 axis, and can be restored in part by the administration of human growth hormone."[2]

IT'S A FACT

People with cancer should not take HGH or peptides.

HGH benefit 3: cheap and effective alternatives

Remember, very few adults will have low growth hormone on the insulin tolerance test or the glucagon stimulation test, and therefore, doctors will not prescribe growth hormone. We can still benefit from peptides. HGH shots are usually extremely pricey. Yes, incredibly effective, but very few can afford it or want to spend their money in that way, especially since peptides usually are so effective.

But as we have already discussed, peptides and amino acid secretagogues are often sufficient to get our pituitary glands pumping out growth hormone again and are relatively inexpensive.

Several different studies have found that to be the case when amino acids arginine and lysine are taken together. One study found that just 1500 mg of each (arginine and lysine) significantly increased human growth hormone levels.[3] In another study, this time of men ranging in age from thirty-two to sixty-four, the men were given 2000 mg of the amino acid glutamine, and just ninety minutes later their human growth hormone levels had increased over 400 percent.[4]

The point is, I'm convinced without question that boosting human growth hormone levels benefits our bodies. In my perspective, many over the age of fifty ought to do this, especially if they are having some of the symptoms of low HGH. The fact that we can all afford it makes it that much better. I suggest starting with amino acids, such as lysine, arginine, or glutamine, if under fifty, which you can get at most health food stores.

THE HORMONE HEALTH ZONE FOR HGH IN ALL OF US

Optimizing your growth hormone levels will ideally happen in conjunction with the optimizing of your other hormone levels. Doing so will maximize the effectiveness of the increased growth hormone levels in your body.

As I have mentioned, the normal range for human growth hormone (HGH) in men is 65–199 ng/mL and in women is 58–175 ng/mL. Because it is such a wide range, we all virtually fit within these parameters. When you are optimizing your growth hormone levels back to what they were when you were in your twenties, I recommend you aim to raise your IGF-1 level, which is the main way to increase growth hormone, to 200–250 ng/mL (sometimes up to 300 ng/mL if you're not experiencing side effects). When you request your insulin-like growth factor 1 (IGF-1) test, it will give you a starting point, and from there you can chart your course to optimize that level to 200–250 ng/mL.

Getting your growth hormone levels up to this level can usually cause several things to happen in your body, including:

- fewer wrinkles
- thicker skin
- fuller hair
- sharper memory
- greater muscle tone and strength
- weight loss
- increased bone strength
- better sleep

If those are not good enough reasons to boost your growth hormone levels, did you know that as we age, our organs shrink and our brains shrink? Higher growth hormone levels will help stop the shrinking and usually help return organs and the brain to their proper sizes. For all of us, the time to start increasing our growth hormone levels is now, especially if we are over fifty years of age.

CONCLUSION

I F YOU WERE to take a moment and list some of the diseases out there, perhaps some of which might even run in your family history, the list would look something like this:

- breast cancer
- heart disease
- high cholesterol
- obesity
- type 2 diabetes
- glaucoma
- prostate cancer
- Hashimoto's
- Alzheimer's
- Parkinson's
- dementia
- fibromyalgia
- osteoporosis
- sarcopenia
- insomnia
- arthritis
- chronic illness (fatigue, depression, pain, and so on)

Odds are, even this short list strikes pretty close to home. If not, the list of symptoms from chapter 3 may do the same. The point is, all these diseases and the long list of symptoms do not necessarily have the power over us that they once had. Why? Because we now have answers! When we optimize our hormone levels, many of these diseases and symptoms can potentially begin to vanish, never to return!

When we get our hormone levels back to the levels they were at when we were in our twenties, our health has a way of drastically improving! When we add a good diet, exercise, nutrition, and a healthy lifestyle (less stress, choose to forgive, walk in peace, and so on) to optimized hormone levels, our bodies respond in incredible ways! That is incredible news!

And because we are talking about *your* life and *your* body, the next step is up to you. Optimizing your hormones with bioidentical hormone replacement therapy is safer, easier, and cheaper than it has ever been. Finding a doctor who will work with you to address the root cause of your symptoms is also much easier than ever. Please refer to the list of websites in appendix F to find this type of doctor.

You may have to travel to find an antiaging or age-management doctor, but those doctors are out there, far more than in years past. Take the time and spend the effort to find a doctor who will work with you. Trust me; it will be worth it! (And when you do find the right doctor, be patient. Start low and go slow.)

Yes, you will probably get some pushback in your desire to find lasting solutions to your symptoms. Conventional medicine takes more of a "patch it" rather than "fix it" approach, and most doctors will view your low or suboptimal hormone levels as "in range" and do nothing about it. Your symptoms will be screaming for an answer, and no prescription, especially not an antidepressant, antianxiety medication, or cholesterol-lowering drug, will help.

In my world medical information doubles every seventy-three days. Unless a doctor is running fast to keep up with the newest and latest advances in the medical world, he is going to be left far behind. Every antiaging doctor who is on the cutting edge of the industry has had to run, study, and work hard to be there.

Doctors who do not keep up naturally drift backward. I've found that most doctors are probably ten or twenty years behind. That means you might be trusting someone who is good but who does not have enough information or the latest information. That's just the way it is in the medical profession.

Look at it another way. Let's say you need to buy a new cell phone, and you walk into a store. There are two attendants behind the counter. One is holding a flip phone, and the other is holding the newest cell phone model. Whom do you trust? Whom do you go to for help? The old flip phone wasn't all that long ago, and I used to have one, but that is the same outdatedness that occurs in the medical world, and even more so.

ADVICE TO FELLOW DOCTORS

If you are a doctor reading this, I suggest that you learn about the power of bioidentical hormone replacement therapy as

quickly as you can and eventually hire several nurse practitio-
ners because your business is going to explode!

Now, I am not blaming the doctors. They are typically overwhelmed
with work, charts, running the business, making ends meet, meeting
quotas, going to meetings, and talking with pharmaceutical reps.
They usually only have ten to fifteen minutes to see you and prescribe
a medication to treat your problem. It is the system, not the doctor,
that is wrong. In truth, it's more of a "disease care system" than it is
a health care system.

What we need is a paradigm shift, a new way of thinking, that seeks
to fix (prevent, stop, and repair) rather than merely patch. As this new
global shift happens (and it is happening!), if doctors and companies
don't keep up, they will be left behind. People are changing. They are
not willing to get on and stay on medications for the rest of their lives.
They are demanding answers that bring freedom, health, and vitality,
not further pain, discomfort, and more negative symptoms.

IT'S A FACT

When you regain your shape, you also regain your self-
confidence, strength, energy, life, vitality, muscles, and a
whole lot more!

Simply put, you as the patient get to choose. It's your body, so your
vote counts the most. You decide how you want to live your life. And
when you do choose to look for answers that fix the problem rather
than patch it, remember that *optimized* hormone levels are the goal
rather than just *balanced* hormone levels. Of course, balanced is
much better than low or suboptimal hormone levels, but only when
your hormone levels are optimized do diseases and symptoms usually melt away.

Hitting the optimized level is many times like a reset button.
Having the hormone function and mental clarity that you did when
you were twenty-five? That is powerful. It is exciting! It is usually a
brand-new start in life!

I have seen so many people begin to feel great again. They get energized, feel full of life, regrow muscle and bone, lose weight, become

disease resistant, and regain their hope. It's almost as if their bodies have been reset to youth. After all, your greatest wealth is your health, so do all you can to optimize it!

To your health, life, and happiness! And one more thing: long life!

TWENTY-ONE-DAY HORMONE HEALTH ZONE CHALLENGE

A s I've mentioned throughout this book, most people can balance their hormones with the bioidentical hormone products I've discussed. But to maximize their effectiveness and go from hormone balance to hormone optimization, a healthy diet, exercise, and a healthy lifestyle are going to be necessary components for most people. One married couple basically took the diet and exercise recommendations from my Keto Zone book (see appendix F) and tweaked them to fit an optimized hormone lifestyle. I've recapped their plan here, and I challenge you to try it for twenty-one days to boost your hormone health. I believe it will really benefit you to do what they did, and when you experience the results for yourself, you'll want to keep it going longer than the twenty-one days as part of your new, healthy life in the hormone health zone.

FOOD OPTIONS

Carbs: Carbs are supposed to be 15 percent of the daily intake (mostly from salads, green vegetables, spices, and herbs), consistent with a ketogenic diet or my Keto Zone Diet.

Fat: Fat is supposed to be 70 percent of daily intake (from fish oil, MCT oil, avocado oil, olive oil, nuts, and small amounts of grass-fed butter, ghee, and cheese).

Proteins: Proteins are supposed to be 15 percent of daily intake (from whole pastured eggs, pastured chicken and turkey, wild fish, and grass-fed meats). Aim for 1 g of protein per 1 kg of body weight.

Their breakfasts rotated but were typically:

- 2–3 fried eggs (in coconut oil, grass-fed butter, or avocado oil) with sliced veggies (tomatoes, mushrooms, spinach), with slices of ham, or with 2–3 turkey bacon strips
- 2- or 3-egg omelet (with spinach, cheese, ham)
- smoothie made with low-sugar almond milk, 1 scoop egg white protein, 1 Tbsp almond butter, 1 Tbsp MCT oil powder or avocado oil, and ¼ cup frozen berries
- coffee with 1–2 Tbsp MCT oil powder and/or 1 Tbsp avocado oil

Their lunches also rotated but typically included:

- salad with 4–6 oz pastured chicken, steak, turkey, or wild salmon, including cucumbers, tomatoes, celery, cheese, and 3–4 Tbsp olive oil/apple cider vinegar dressing
- chicken or tongol tuna salad with 2–3 Tbsp olive-oil- or avocado-oil-based mayo and celery, chives, onions, pickles, jalapeño cream cheese, and nuts (pecans, almonds, or walnuts)
- hamburger wrapped in romaine lettuce leaves with tomato, avocado, salt, and pepper with 2–3 Tbsp avocado-oil mayonnaise

Dinners also rotated but were often:

- grilled fish or shrimp with green beans, asparagus, or broccoli cooked in 1–2 Tbsp grass-fed butter and 1–2 Tbsp avocado oil or olive oil
- grilled steak or chicken with veggies sautéed in 2 Tbsp olive oil or salad tossed with 2–4 Tbsp avocado oil or olive oil and apple cider vinegar
- stir-fried beef, shrimp, or chicken with broccoli, green beans, cabbage, bok choy, onion, peppers, garlic, and

mushrooms with 1–2 Tbsp grass-fed butter and 1–2 Tbsp avocado oil

- grilled salmon over raw spinach with Himalayan salt, pepper, lemon, minced garlic, and 2–3 Tbsp olive oil on top

Snacks:

- celery with guacamole and salsa
- nuts (macadamia, pecans, almonds, walnuts), salt and vinegar peanuts, and garlic and onion macadamia nuts
- only Keto Zone-friendly desserts (See www.ketozone.com.)
- sunflower and pumpkin seeds
- jalapeño cream cheese and celery
- peanut butter or almond butter and cucumber slices

Supplements:

- multivitamin with iodine included
- fish oil
- probiotics
- vitamin D_3

BEVERAGES

- alkaline or sparkling water and may add lemon or lime wedges
- coffee, especially keto coffee with MCT oil powder (See www.ketozone.com.)
- green tea
- low-sugar coconut or almond milk

EXERCISE OPTIONS

They created a short workout that built muscle as well as gave them sufficient cardio exercise, and that worked with their busy schedules. It included:

- lifting weights (barbells) for about ten to twenty minutes (they had separate barbells) that exercised numerous muscle groups, including their arms, shoulders, backs, and thighs, three times each set

- planking for one minute a day, five days a week (To plank, assume the pushup position with back and neck and legs flat like a plank. Maintain that position for one minute and breathe. You can start on your knees if your strength isn't built up to a full plank position.)

- walking briskly for thirty minutes in the evenings five times a week

- biking through a local park for thirty minutes on weekends or recumbent bike for thirty minutes five days a week

LIFESTYLE OPTIONS

They found several ways to decrease the stresses in their lives, including practicing better communication with each other, being quicker to forgive and let go of offenses, choosing to not let stress eat away at them, reading the Bible upon awakening in the morning and before bed, maintaining a time of prayer, meditation, and reading every morning, and ten belly laughs every day. They watched old Carol Burnett shows each night and got plenty of belly laughter that way. All of this helped strengthen their adrenal glands.

21-DAY CHALLENGE

What about you? Try the above for twenty-one days. Odds are, you will feel better, be mentally sharper, have less stress, and perhaps even lose some weight.

Keep it up! Turn the twenty-one-day challenge into a lifetime. Tweak it. Change it up. It's your body. You can enjoy it for the rest of your life! For more helpful information on how to eat a ketogenic diet as summarized in this challenge, please refer to my book *Dr. Colbert's Keto Zone Diet* and my new Keto Zone cookbook.

APPENDIX B

THE EIGHT PILLARS OF HEALTH

USED TO BELIEVE there were seven pillars of health. My first *New York Times* best seller was even titled *The Seven Pillars of Health*. It turns out, I now believe there are eight pillars! Here they are:

Pillar 1: have an adequate intake of water. Most people don't drink enough water. Distilled or reverse osmosis water is acidic. I recommend alkaline water. It's critical for the cells to function optimally.

Pillar 2: get adequate sleep. That means seven to eight hours a night. Here is how you can tell if you get adequate sleep. Do you awaken refreshed in the morning? If not, then you are not getting adequate sleep. It is critical for restoring your body's function. At night is when our bodies repair most tissues and organs. Sleep is also critical for helping to restore your adrenal glands as well as keeping your body healthy, keeping your immune system strong, and helping prevent weight gain to obesity. The term *beauty sleep* is absolutely correct because sleep also helps optimize your growth hormone levels that keep you looking young. (You can refer to my book *The Ultimate Sleep Guide* for more information.)

Pillar 3: cope with stress. Being able to handle the stresses of life is critical. This is such an important issue that I wrote an entire book on it (*Stress Less*). Stress is probably the greatest killer today. It invites every disease into the body. Learning to cope with, handle, avoid, and deal with stress is vital.

Pillar 4: eat living foods versus dead foods. Living foods bring life, but processed foods invite disease and eventually death into your body. I discovered the importance of anti-inflammatory and ketogenic diet, and that is all about living foods. (I wrote *Let Food Be Your Medicine* and *Dr. Colbert's Keto Zone Diet* to address those two very real issues.) We unknowingly invite most diseases into our bodies by choosing inflammatory foods, such as sugar, processed foods, excessive starches, inflammatory fats, and excessive carbohydrates and processed meats. (Other books I've written on this topic are *Eat This and Live!* and *Reversing Inflammation*.)

Pillar 5: supplement. We usually do not get adequate nutrition from the foods we eat, so everyone requires certain supplements in order to help prevent disease. If our food doesn't supply the nutrition we need, then the only way to get it is through supplementation. A good multivitamin is a good place to begin, but other supplements are most likely required. (Refer to my book *Dr. Colbert's Guide to Vitamins and Supplements* for helpful information on choosing the right supplements.)

Pillar 6: detoxify. On a regular basis we need to rid our bodies of toxins that we are exposed to on a daily basis. It is important to detox the colon, liver, and key organs of elimination. Detox regularly with nutrients, certain detoxifying foods, alkaline water, and an infrared sauna. (I've written a book called *Toxic Relief* that provides a wealth of information on this topic.)

Pillar 7: exercise. Regular exercise is extremely important in maintaining health. Exercises that strengthen muscles are vital, as are core exercises such as planks, aerobic exercise, and postural exercises. (I've outlined some great exercise recommendations in my book *Get Fit and Live!*)

Pillar 8: optimize your hormone levels. I have found nothing so beneficial to your body's overall health and rejuvenation as optimizing hormone levels. For optimal health, optimizing hormone levels is a necessity. That's the newest pillar and why I've written this important book.

And there you have it. With the eight pillars of health at work in your body (your temple), you have all the elements in place for a long, healthy, enjoyable life!

APPENDIX C

NORMAL HORMONE RANGES AT A GLANCE

THE MAIN HORMONES that need to be tested and then optimized in your body include total testosterone, free testosterone, TSH, free T3, free T4, TPO, rT3, estradiol, progesterone (for women), FSH (for women), and IFG-1. Here's a quick reference guide for the normal range for each of these hormones, as stated by blood-testing companies such as LabCorp or Quest Diagnostics, along with what I recommend as optimized hormone level ranges.

HORMONE	RANGE	OPTIMIZED
Total testosterone (men)	264–916 ng/dL	900–1100 ng/dL
Total testosterone (women)	15–70 ng/dL	60–70 ng/dL and higher for those with osteoporosis or sarcopenia (see chapter 10)
Free testosterone (men)	46–224 pg/mL	150–224 pg/mL
Free testosterone (women)	0.2–5.0 pg/mL (ages 18–69), 0.3–5.0 pg/mL (ages 70–89)	7–10 pg/mL
TSH	0.45 – 4.5 µIU/mL	0.1–1.0 µIU/L or lower
Free T3	2.0–4.4 pg/mL	3.5–4.4 pg/mL
Free T4	0.8–1.8 ng/dL	1.2–1.8 ng/dL
rT3	less than 15 ng/dl	less than 15 ng/dl
Antibodies—TPOAbs or TGAbs	10–20 IU/mL	less than 10 IU/mL
FSH	A young woman in mid cycle has a FSH of 4.5–23 IU/L	less than 23 IU/L
Estradiol (men)	20–70 pg/mL	20–50 pg/mL

HORMONE	RANGE	OPTIMIZED
Estradiol (women)	2-to-1 ratio estradiol over estrone	More than 2-to-1 ratio estradiol over estrone
Progesterone (women)	0.1–25 ng/mL	10–20 ng/mL
Progesterone (men)	0.0–0.5 ng/mL	n/a
IFG–1	Ages 51–60: 87–225 ng/mL (men), 92–190 ng/mL (women) Ages 61–70: 75–228 ng/mL (men), 87–178 ng/mL (women) Ages: 71–80: 31–187 ng/mL (men), 25–171 ng/mL (women) Ages 81–88: 68–157 ng/mL (men), 31–162 ng/mL (women)	200–250 ng/mL

HOW TO MAXIMIZE YOUR T4-TO-T3 CONVERSION

THE PROCESS OF raising your active free T3 thyroid hormone level is not that complicated, and when you do it, you will notice the effects, and usually immediately. You increase your active free T3 levels by maximizing the T4-to-T3 conversion process through:

- aerobic exercise
- increased lean body mass
- optimized hormone levels
- adding T3 to your current regimen of T4
- switching to a T4 and T3 combination medication
- supplements such as B vitamins, vitamin D, vitamin C, iodine, ashwagandha, selenium, magnesium, zinc, and glutathione (an amino acid)
- decreasing stress
- getting adequate, quality sleep, usually seven to eight hours a night

ADDITIONAL TIPS

- Your body needs glucagon, insulin, melatonin, testosterone, human growth hormone (HGH), and cortisol to properly convert T4 to T3. If these are too low or if insulin is too high, conversion isn't happening as it should.[1]

- Iron deficiency and low ferritin levels lead to poor T4-to-T3 conversion. Coffee, tea, acid blockers, antacids, and blood pressure medications are the top causes of iron depletion in your body.[2]

- I have found that most of my patients with thyroid issues see significant improvement when they reduce gluten or go gluten-free. Do they suffer from celiac disease? Not likely, but the gluten of today has a way of inflaming our bodies and especially our GI tract, and that may eventually affect the thyroid.

- In my practice I see gluten intolerance or gluten sensitivity in a large percentage of my thyroid patients, and estimates are 10–14 percent of Hashimoto's thyroiditis patients have celiac disease.[3] I ask most of my Hashimoto's patients to go gluten-free for three months to see if it helps. Almost everyone who does it rarely goes back to eating gluten because his or her symptoms usually improve: IBS improves or goes away; fatigue and brain fog usually improve; and TPO antibodies usually come down. Getting off gluten is for many the biggest breakthrough in overcoming their thyroid symptoms.

The most common things that decrease your T3 levels by decreasing your T4-to-T3 conversion process are:

- stress (Stress by itself is enough to decrease your active free T3; stress also impedes conversion of T4 to T3.)
- inflammation from food, sickness, or allergies
- nutrient deficiencies
- high cortisol levels
- chronic sickness
- lack of exercise
- aging
- certain prescribed medications, especially lithium, beta-blockers, birth control pills, and glucocorticoids

- hormone disruptors
- low testosterone levels

Approximately 90 percent of the thyroid hormone your body produces is the inactive T4, and only about 7 percent is the active T3. That is the norm for all of us. The liver is where most of the T4 is processed and converted to T3. Most of us can convert about 40 percent of the T4 our bodies make to T3. Interestingly about 20 percent of the total is converted in our gastrointestinal tract, which means if we have a healthy gut, we are utilizing that 20 percent, but if we have an unhealthy gut, we are missing 20 percent of the most useful thyroid hormone, T3, and that is not good!

The higher your free T3 hormone level, the more T4-to-T3 conversion is taking place in your body, and that results in a healthier body. How you feel and your symptoms, or lack of symptoms, will support this. You want your optimized thyroid levels (pushed to the upper or lower ranges) to be close to these:

- free T3: 3.5–4.4 pg/mL
- free T4: 1.2–1.8 ng/dL (optional)
- TSH: 0.1–1.0 µIU/L or lower
- rT3: less than 15 ng/dL (based on the 20-to-1 ratio)
- antibodies: TPOAb or TGAb: less than 10 IU/mL (optional)
- free T3-to-rT3 ratio: 20 to 1 or greater

These are the most important numbers to know, track, and manage with your thyroid, but in particular your free T3 and rT3 are the numbers to watch. Therefore, testing for free T3 and rT3 is considered to be critical when optimizing hormone levels. Most doctors do not even test for these two, so be sure that you request them.

HOW TO LOWER YOUR RT3 LEVELS

L OWERING YOUR BODY's rT3 begins by taking T3 (liothyronine). I usually start with 2.5–5 mcg of liothyronine twice a day. You don't need any more T4, as you already have T4 in excess, so taking T3 only automatically starts lowering your T4 levels, which lowers your rT3 as well.

Increase the dosage slowly every three or four days by 2.5–5 mcg per dose until you are at 25 mcg twice a day, and then stay at that level for about three months. Monitor your pulse two to three times each day along the way. Make sure your pulse does not go over 100 while resting or that you have no palpitations or irregular heartbeats. If your pulse goes over 100 at rest, decrease your dose to the dose when your pulse was less than 100. If your symptoms subside and your pulse normalizes, stay at that dose for one week, and then only increase the dose by 2.5 mcg or less. If a rapid heart rate occurs again, stay at the lower dosage that was without symptoms. Follow up with a physician if palpitations, elevated pulse, or irregular heart rate continues after you have lowered the dose or stopped the thyroid.

Take a multivitamin as well as the supplement selenium (100–200 mg once per day). Eating according to the Keto Zone diet (see appendix F) is recommended, as is an exercise program that uses aerobic exercise, weights, and core exercises. Use caution and consult your age management physician if you are over sixty or have a history of atrial fibrillation, arrhythmia, coronary artery disease, congestive heart failure, or any form of heart disease.

What lowers your rT3 levels:

- Vitamin A (4000 IU daily)
- Iodine (150 mcg daily)

- Iron (men: 8 mg; women: 18 mg to menopause, 8 mg after menopause, daily. Most men do not need iron.)
- Selenium (100–200 mcg a day)
- Decrease alcohol consumption.
- Stop smoking.
- Take liver support supplements, such as NAC, glutathione, Max One, or milk thistle.
- Decrease sugar intake.
- Take T3 only.
- Boost adrenal function with supplements.
- Decrease stress.
- Stop using artificial sweeteners.
- Minimize processed foods.
- Avoid refined vegetable oils and trans fats.

The more rT3 your body creates, the more thyroid issues you will probably have. So you want your rT3 levels to be at the low end of normal. As a reminder, the rT3 number you want to aim for is less than 15 ng/dL. Decreasing rT3 as much as possible will pay big dividends to your overall health.

APPENDIX F

SUPPLEMENTS AND RESOURCES

KETO ZONE SUPPLEMENTS AT KETOZONE.COM OR DRCOLBERT.COM

Keto Zone MCT oil powder (coconut, French vanilla, and hazelnut)

Keto Zone instant ketones

Keto Zone Fat-Zyme

Keto Zone collagen

DIVINE HEALTH NUTRITIONAL PRODUCTS AT DRCOLBERT.COM

Green supreme food

Red supreme food

Iced krill

Enhanced multivitamin

Living chia

HORMONE HEALTH ZONE PRODUCTS AT DRCOLBERT.COM

- Testosterone zone (provides clinically studied ingredients, including synergistic nutrients and herbs that boost free testosterone levels)
- Hormone zone (contains DIM and synergistic nutrients that provide hormone support for men and women)
- Thyroid zone (a blend of nutrients and herbs designed specifically to provide thyroid support)

LAB TESTING

Hormone health zone blood panel

> For men: TSH, free T3, total and free testosterone, SHBG, estradiol, rT3, TPO, and PSA

> For women: TSH, free T3, total and free testosterone, estradiol, rT3, TPO, FSH, and progesterone level

Divine health panel

> For men: all hormone tests for men, and CMP, CBC, HbA1C, CRP, 25OHD3 level, B_{12} level, urinalysis, and lipid panel

> For women: all hormone tests for women and additional tests above

> Adrenal testing (DiagnosTechs Adrenal Panel) at diagnostechs .com

> DHEAS level (blood test)

> Salivary cortisol testing at 8:00 a.m., noon, 4:00 p.m., and 8:00 p.m.

Physician locator

> worldhealth.net

> agemanagement.org

> biotemedical.com

> agemed.org

> brodabarnes.org

THE TEN MOST COMMON
ENDOCRINE DISRUPTORS[1]

SOMETIMES WHAT YOU don't know and can't see can actually hurt you. That is certainly the case with endocrine (hormone) disruptors. Here are the ten most common disruptors, as compiled by the Environmental Working Group, and what you can do to avoid them.

1. BPA (bisphenol A): Statistics show that almost all of us have BPA in our bodies, which has been found to be linked to decreased fertility, heart disease, obesity, breast and other cancers, and much more. It is most often found in the lining of metal cans, in plastic containers, and in most cash register receipts. HOW TO AVOID: If you can't buy fresh or frozen, buy food in glass jars rather than canned food. Store food in non-plastic containers, and don't touch receipts.

2. Dioxins: These leftovers from many industrial processing plants are found to lower sperm counts in men and are carcinogenic (cancer causing). They also accumulate and over time can cause real damage, even to babies in the womb. HOW TO AVOID: Dioxins are in most of the fatty animal products we eat, so decreasing intake of meats, eggs, cheese, butter, cream, and so on, can help decrease dioxins.

3. Atrazine: This is the second–most widely used weed killer and is the most common chemical contaminant in the US water supply. It has been found to turn male frogs into female frogs! In animals, breast cancer, delayed puberty, and prostate issues are connected to atrazine exposure. HOW TO AVOID: Buying organic produce can help, but the biggest way to decrease atrazine exposure is to get a water filter in your home.

4. Phthalates: Cell damage in the testes is the result of phthalate accumulation in your body. Birth defects in male reproductive tissues, low sperm count, thyroid issues, and many other problems are linked to

phthalate exposure. HOW TO AVOID: Watch out for personal care products (with "fragrance" listed) that contain phthalates. Do not microwave food or beverages in plastic containers. Do not store food in plastic containers or bags.

5. Perchlorate: This endocrine disruptor directly affects your thyroid by competing with iodine, and that affects your metabolism, brain, and organs. HOW TO AVOID: It's usually in the water, so a good water filter will do the trick. Also, iodine supplementation can help reduce the effects of perchlorate in your body.

6. Polybrominated diphenyl ethers (PBDEs) used as fire retardants: These chemicals also have a negative impact on your thyroid hormones. PBDEs have been phased out, but they linger in the environment everywhere. HOW TO AVOID: Decreasing the dust in your house by using a vacuum that has a HEPA filter will help.

7. Mercury: This endocrine disruptor can cause brain damage with unborn children because it accumulates in the mother's body. Often found in seafood, it is hard to avoid. HOW TO AVOID: Choose fish that are low in mercury, such as wild salmon, halibut, anchovies, perch, pollack, sole, tilapia, trout, herring, sardines, tuna (tongol), and flounder.

8. Perfluorochemicals (PFCs): Virtually all of us (99 percent) have these chemicals in our bodies, and they accumulate steadily. Again, they decrease thyroid hormones and cause many issues (kidney disease, high cholesterol, low birth weight, low sperm count, and more). HOW TO AVOID: PFCs are often found in nonstick pans and stain- and water-resistant coatings, so avoiding those is your best defense.

9. Organophosphate pesticides: These pesticides are used to kill insects, but they also affect humans by lowering our testosterone and thyroid hormone levels. HOW TO AVOID: Buying organic produce can help.

10. Glycol ethers: These are solvents found in paints and cleaning products, and even in some cosmetics. They can damage unborn children and decrease fertility in men by lowering sperm counts. HOW TO AVOID: Use natural cleaning alternatives such as vinegar and baking soda, and avoid products with glycol ethers, such as 2-butoxyethanol (EGBE) and methoxydiglycol (DEBME).

We might not be able to avoid all these endocrine disruptors, but if we can minimize our exposure, we are also reducing the accumulation in our bodies. Over time this will be highly beneficial to your health!

NOTES

INTRODUCTION

1. "Adult Obesity Facts," Centers for Disease Control and Prevention, accessed September 17, 2018, https://www.cdc.gov/obesity/data/adult .html.
2. "A Snapshot: Diabetes in the United States," Centers for Disease Control and Prevention, accessed September 17, 2018, https://www.cdc .gov/diabetes/library/socialMedia/infographics.html.
3. "Heart Disease Facts," Centers for Disease Control and Prevention, accessed September 17, 2018, https://www.cdc.gov/heartdisease/facts. htm.
4. "Alzheimer's Disease," Centers for Disease Control and Prevention, accessed September 17, 2018, https://www.cdc.gov/aging/aginginfo /alzheimers.htm.
5. "Preventable Adverse Drug Reactions: A Focus on Drug Interactions," US Food and Drug Administration, accessed September 17, 2018, https://www.fda.gov/drugs/developmentapprovalprocess /developmentresources/druginteractionslabeling/ucm110632.htm.
6. Kathy C. Maupin, *The Secret Female Hormone* (Carlsbad, CA: Hay House, 2014), 83; L. M. Alderson and M. J. Baum, "Differential Effects of Gonadal Steroids on Dopamine Metabolism in Mesolimbic and Nigro-Striatal Pathways of Male Rat Brain," *Brain Research* 218, no. 1-2 (August 10, 1981): 189–206, https://www.ncbi.nlm.nih.gov/pubmed /7272735.

CHAPTER 1

1. "Nearly 7 in 10 Americans Take Prescription Drugs, Mayo Clinic, Olmsted Medical Center Find," Mayo Clinic, June 19, 2013, https:// newsnetwork.mayoclinic.org/discussion/nearly-7-in-10-americans-take-prescription-drugs mayo clinic-olmsted-medical-center-find/.

CHAPTER 2

1. Troy Brown, "The 10 Most-Prescribed and Top-Selling Medications," WebMD, accessed September 18, 2018, https://www.webmd.com/drug-medication/news/20150508/most-prescribed-top-selling-drugs.
2. Erika Schwartz, *The New Hormone Solution* (Brentwood, TN: Post Hill Press, 2017), 185.

3. C. E. Wood et al., "Effects of Estradiol With Micronized Progesterone or Medroxyprogesterone Acetate on Risk Markers for Breast Cancer in Postmenopausal Monkeys," *Breast Cancer Research and Treatment* 101, no. 2 (January 2007): 125–34, https://doi.org/10.1007/s10549-006-9276-y; Y. Liang et al., "Synthetic Progestins Induce Growth and Metastasis of BT-474 Human Breast Cancer Xenografts in Nude Mice," *Menopause* 17, no. 5 (September–October 2010): 1040–7, https://doi.org/10.1097/gme.0b013e3181d3dd0c; K. Ory et al., "Apoptosis Inhibition Mediated by Medroxyprogesterone Acetate Treatment of Breast Cancer Cell Lines," *Breast Cancer Research and Treatment* 68, no. 3 (August 2001): 187–98, https://www.ncbi.nlm.nih.gov/pubmed/11727956.

4. D. Murkes et al., "Effects of Percutaneous Estradiol-Oral Progesterone Versus Oral Conjugated Equine Estrogens-Medroxyprogesterone Acetate on Breast Cell Proliferation and Bcl-2 Protein in Healthy Women," *Fertility and Sterility* 95, no. 3 (March 1, 2011): 1188–91, https://doi.org/10.1016/j.fertnstert.2010.09.062; C. E. Wood, "Transcriptional Profiles of Progestogen Effects in the Postmenopausal Breast," *Breast Cancer Research and Treatment* 114, no. 2 (March 2009): 233–42, https://doi.org/10.1007/s10549-008-0003-8; H. Neubauer et al., "Overexpression of Progesterone Receptor Membrane Component 1: Possible Mechanism for Increased Breast Cancer Risk With Norethisterone in Hormone Therapy," *Menopause* 20, no. 5 (May 2013): 504–10, https://doi.org/10.1097/GME.0b013e3182755c97; D. Murkes et al., "Percutaneous Estradiol/Oral Micronized Progesterone Has Less-Adverse Effects and Different Gene Regulations Than Oral Conjugated Equine Estrogens/Medroxyprogesterone Acetate in the Breasts of Healthy Women in Vivo," *Gynecological Endocrinology* 28, no. 2 (October 2012): 12–15, https://doi.org/10.3109/09513590.2012.706670; K. J. Chang et al., "Influences of Percutaneous Administration of Estradiol and Progesterone on Human Breast Epithelial Cell Cycle in Vivo," *Fertility and Sterility* 63, no. 4 (April 1995): 785–91, https://www.ncbi.nlm.nih.gov/pubmed/7890063; C. E. Wood et al., "Effects of Estradiol," 125–34.

5. L. A. Pratt, D. J. Brody, and Q. Gu, "Antidepressant Use in Persons Aged 12 and Over: United States, 2005–2008," NCHS data brief, no. 76, Hyattsville, MD: National Center for Health Statistics, 2011.

6. Loretta Lanphier, "1 in 4 Women on Antidepressant Drugs for Stress, Depression, Anxiety," The Best Years in Life, accessed September 18, 2018, http://www.tbyil.com/1_in_4_Women_on_Antidepressant_Drugs_Loretta_Lanphier.htm.

7. "Cholesterol," Centers for Disease Control and Prevention, accessed September 18, 2018, https://www.cdc.gov/cholesterol/index.htm.

8. Suzy Cohen, *Thyroid Healthy* (Louisiana: Dear Pharmacist Inc., 2014), 17.

9. Marcia L. Stefanick, et al., "Effects of Conjugated Equine Estrogens on Breast Cancer and Mammography Screening in Postmenopausal Women With Hysterectomy," *Journal of the American Medical Association* 295, no. 14 (2006): 1647–1657, https://doi.org/10.1001/jama.295.14.1647; A. Patrick Schneider et al., "The Breast Cancer Epidemic: 10 Facts," *Linacre Quarterly* 81, no. 3 (August 2014): 244–77, https://doi.org/10.1179/2050854914Y.0000000027.

10. Gary Donovitz, *Age Healthier, Live Happier* (Florida: Celebrity Press, 2015), 77.

11. Philip M. Sarrel et al., "The Mortality Toll of Estrogen Avoidance: An Analysis of Excess Deaths Among Hysterectomized Women Aged 50 to 59 Years," *American Journal of Public Health* 103, no. 9 (September 2013): 1583–8, https://doi.org/10.2105/AJPH.2013.301295.

12. Schwartz, *The New Hormone Solution*, 5.

13. Jay Campbell and Jim Brown, *The Testosterone Optimization Therapy Bible* (Pasadena, California: Best Seller Publishing, 2018), 25.

14. Shehzad Basaria et al., "Adverse Events Associated With Testosterone Administration," *New England Journal of Medicine* 363 (July 8, 2010): 109–22, https://doi.org/10.1056/NEJMoa1000485.

15. Rebecca Vigen et al., "Association of Testosterone Therapy With Mortality, Myocardial Infarction, and Stroke in Men With Low Testosterone Levels," *Journal of the American Medical Association* 310, no. 17 (November 2013): 1829–36, https://doi.org/10.1001/jama.2013.280386.

16. "Comment & Response: Deaths and Cardiovascular Events in Men Receiving Testosterone," *Journal of the American Medical Association* 311, no. 9 (March 5, 2014): 961–5, http://smsna.org/V1/images/JAMA/letters%20to%20the%20Editors%20accepted%20by%20JAMA%20%20regarding%20Vegin%20et%20al%20paper.pdf; Arthi Thirumalai, Katya B. Rubinow, and Stephanie T. Page, "An Update on Testosterone, HDL and Cardiovascular Risk in Men," *Journal of Clinical Lipidology* 10, no. 3 (2015): 251–58, https://www.ncbi.nlm.nih.gov/pmc/articles/PMC4527564/; Abdulmaged M. Traish, "Testosterone Therapy in Men With Testosterone Deficiency: Are the Benefits and Cardiovascular Risks Real or Imagined?," *American Journal of Physiology* 311, no. 3 (September 2016), https://doi.org/10.1152/ajpregu.00174.2016.

17. C. J. Malkin et al., "Low Serum Testosterone and Increased Mortality in Men With Coronary Heart Disease," *Heart*, 96, no. 22 (November 2010): 1821–5, https://dx.doi.org/10.1136/hrt2010.195412.

18. Rishi Sharma et al., "Normalization of Testosterone Level is Associated With Reduced Incidence of Myocardial Infarction and Mortality in Men," *European Heart Journal* 36, no. 40 (October 21, 2015): 2706–15, https://doi.org/10.1093/eurheartj/ehv346.

19. Abraham Morgentaler, *Testosterone for Life* (New York: McGraw-Hill, 2008), 134.

20. G. M. Rosano et al., "Natural Progesterone, but Not Medroxyprogesterone Acetate, Enhances the Beneficial Effect of Estrogen on Exercise-Induced Myocardial Ischemia in Postmenopausal Women," *Journal of the American College of Cardiology* 36, no. 7 (December 2000): 2154–9, https://doi.org/10.1016/S0735-1097(00)01007-X; A. Fournier, F. Berrino, and F. Clavel-Chapelon, "Unequal Risks for Breast Cancer Associated With Different Hormone Replacement Therapies: Results From the E3N Cohort Study," *Breast Cancer Research and Treatment* 107, no. 1 (January 2008): 103–11, https://doi.org/10.1007/s10549-007-9523-x; K. Holtorf, "The Bioidentical Hormone Debate: Are Bioidentical Hormones (Estradiol, Estriol, and Progesterone) Safer or More Efficacious Than Commonly Used Synthetic Versions in Hormone Replacement Therapy?," *Postgraduate Medicine* 121, no. 1 (January 2009): 73–85, https://doi.org/10.3810/pgm.2009.01.1949; Murkes et al., "Effects of Percutaneous Estradiol-Oral Progesterone Versus Oral Conjugated Equine Estrogens-Medroxyprogesterone Acetate on Breast Cell Proliferation and Bcl-2 Protein in Healthy Women."

21. L. Xu et al., "Testosterone Therapy and Cardiovascular Events Among Men: A Systematic Review and Meta-Analysis of Placebo-Controlled Randomized Trials," *BMC Medicine* 11 (April 2013): 108, https://doi.org/10.1186/1741-7015-11-108.

22. G. K. Gouras et al., "Testosterone Reduces Neuronal Secretion of Alzheimer's β-amyloid Peptides," *Proceedings of the National Academy of Sciences of the United States of America* 97, no. 3 (February 1, 2000): 1202–5, https://www.ncbi.nlm.nih.gov/pmc/articles/PMC15568/.

23. D. Lim et al., "Can Testosterone Replacement Decrease the Memory Problem of Old Age?," *Medical Hypotheses* 60, no. 6 (June 2003): 893–6, https://www.ncbi.nlm.nih.gov/pubmed/12699720.

Chapter 3

1. "Adult Obesity Facts," Centers for Disease Control and Prevention, accessed September 26, 2018, https://www.cdc.gov/obesity/data/adult.html.

2. World Economic Forum and the Harvard School of Public Health, "The Global Economic Burden of Non-communicable Diseases," September 2011, http://www3.weforum.org/docs/WEF_Harvard_HE_GlobalEconomicBurdenNonCommunicableDiseases_2011.pdf.

3. A. Carle et al., "Epidemiology of Subtypes of Hypothyroidism in Denmark," *European Journal of Endocrinology* 154, no. 1 (January 2006): 21–8, https://doi.org/10.1530/eje.1.02068.

Chapter 4

1. Izabella Wentz, *Hashimoto's Thyroiditis: Lifestyle Interventions for Finding and Treating the Root Cause* (Wentz LLC, 2013), 51.
2. Wentz, *Hashimoto's Thyroiditis*, 23.
3. Philip Shabecoff, *Earth Rising: American Environmentalism in the 21st Century* (Island Press, 2001), 149, https://www.amazon.com /Earth-Rising-American-Environmentalism-Century/dp/1559635843.
4. "Toxic Chemicals Found in Minority Cord Blood," EWG, December 2, 2009, https://www.ewg.org/news/news-releases/2009/12/02 /toxic-chemicals-found-minority-cord-blood#.W3HMm9JKgdU.
5. "Testosterone Week: The Declining Virility of Men and the Importance of T," The Art of Manliness, accessed September 26, 2018, https://www.artofmanliness.com/articles/testosterone-week-intro/; Thomas G. Travison et al., "A Population-Level Decline in Serum Testosterone Levels in American Men," *Journal of Clinical Endocrinology & Metabolism* 92, no. 1 (January 1, 2007): 196–202, https://doi.org/10.1210/jc.2006-1375.
6. Vanessa McMains, "Johns Hopkins Study Suggests Medical Errors Are Third-Leading Cause of Death in U.S.," Johns Hopkins University, May 3, 2016, https://hub.jhu.edu/2016/05/03/medical-errors -third-leading-cause-of-death/.
7. Brown, "The 10 Most-Prescribed and Top-Selling Medications."
8. Mayo Clinic staff, "Statin Side Effects: Weigh the Benefits and Risks," Mayo Clinic, accessed September 26, 2018, www.mayoclinic.org /statin-side-effects/art-20046013.
9. "Assessing and Managing Chemicals Under TSCA: Risk Management for Bisphenol A (BPA)," US Environmental Protection Agency, accessed September 26, 2018, https://www.epa.gov/assessing -and-managing-chemicals-under-tsca/risk-management-bisphenol-bpa.
10. P. Alonso-Magdalena, I. Quesada, and A. Nadal, "Endocrine Disruptors in the Etiology of Type 2 Diabetes Mellitus," *Nature Reviews Endocrinology* 7, no. 6 (April 5, 2011): 346–53, https://doi. org/10.1038/nrendo.2011.56.
11. J. L. Carwile and K. B. Michels, "Urinary Bisphenol A and Obesity: NHANES 2003–2006," *Environmental Research* 111, no. 6 (August 2011): 825–30, https://doi.org/10.1016/j.envres.2011.05.014.
12. F. S. vom Saal, "The Estrogenic Endocrine Disrupting Chemical Bisphenol A (BPA) and Obesity," *Molecular and Cellular Endocrinology* 354, no. 1–2 (May 6, 2012): 74–84, https://doi. org/10.1016/j.mce.2012.01.001.
13. L. N. Vandenberg, "Exposure to Bisphenol A in Canada: Invoking the Precautionary Principle," *CMAJ* 183, no. 11 (August 9, 2011): 1265–70, https://doi.org/10.1503/cmaj.101408.
14. Joseph Mercola, "10 Sources of Endocrine Disruptors and How to Avoid Them," Mercola, July 15, 2015, https://articles.mercola

.com/sites/articles/archive/2015/07/15/10-common-sources-endocrine
-disruptors.aspx.

15. S. Biedermann, P. Tschudin, and K. Grob, "Transfer of Bisphenol A From Thermal Printer Paper to the Skin," *Analytical and Bioanalytical Chemistry* 398, no. 1 (September 2010): 571–76, https://doi.org/10.1007/s00216-010-3936-9.

16. "High Levels of Bisphenol A in Paper Currencies From Several Countries, and Implications for Dermal Exposure," *Environmental Science & Technology* 45, no. 16 (July 11, 2011): 6761–8, https://doi.org/10.1021/es200977t.

17. Sara Goodman, "Tests Find More Than 200 Chemicals in Newborn Umbilical Cord Blood," *Scientific American*, December 2, 2009, https://www.scientificamerican.com/article/newborn-babies-chemicals-exposure-bpa/; D. Li et al., "Occupational Exposure to Bisphenol-A (BPA) and the Risk of Self-Reported Male Sexual Dysfunction," *Human Reproduction* 25, no. 2 (February 1, 2010): 519–27, https://doi.org/10.1093/humrep/dep381.

18. Sushil K. Khetan, *Endocrine Disruptors in the Environment* (New Jersey: John Wiley & Sons Inc., 2014), 92.

19. Mikaela Conley, "Is Chemical in Plastic Robbing Men of Sex Appeal?," ABC News, June 28, 2011, https://abcnews.go.com/Health/plastic-compound-bpa-undermine-masculinity/story?id=13940540.

20. Khetan, *Endocrine Disruptors in the Environment*, 73.

21. K. K. Barnes, "A National Reconnaissance of Pharmaceuticals and Other Organic Wastewater Contaminants in the United States—1) Groundwater," *Science of the Total Environment* 402, no. 2–3 (September 1, 2008), 192-200, https://doi.org/10.1016/j.scitotenv.2008.04.028.

22. F. Brucker-Davis et al, "Genetic and Clinical Features of 42 Kindreds With Resistance to Thyroid Hormone. The National Institutes of Health Prospective Study," *Annals of Internal Medicine* 123, no. 8 (1995): 572–83, https://www.ncbi.nlm.nih.gov/pubmed/7677297.

23. Wentz, *Hashimoto's Thyroiditis*, 89.

24. "Why Your Sofa May Harm Your Health," *Guardian*, accessed September 27, 2018, https://www.theguardian.com/science/2010/jan/21/sofas-carpets-pans-thyroid-disease.

25. Wentz, *Hashimoto's Thyroiditis*, 83.

26. Wentz, *Hashimoto's Thyroiditis*, 89.

27. Nelson Vergel, *Testosterone: A Man's Guide* (Texas: Milestones Publishing, 2011), 84.

28. Hagai Levine et al., "Temporal Trends in Sperm Count: a Systematic Review and Meta-Regression Analysis," *Human Reproduction Update* 23, no. 6 (November 1, 2017): 646–59, https://doi.org/10.1093/humupd/dmx022.

Chapter 5

1. "Landmark Study Defines Normal Ranges for Testosterone Levels," Endocrine Society, January 10, 2017, https://www.endocrine.org/news-room/current-press-releases/landmark-study-defines-normal-ranges-for-testosterone-levels; Jeff Minerd, "Normal Range Redefined for Young Men's Testosterone—264–916 ng/dL Is Now the Standard for Ages 19–39," *MedPage Today*, January 12, 2017, https://www.medpagetoday.com/endocrinology/generalendocrinology/62499.
2. "Triiodothyronine (T3), Free," LabCorp, accessed October 23, 2018, https://www.labcorp.com/test-menu/36151/triiodothyronine-tsub3-sub-free.
3. J. Axelsson et al., "Effects of Acutely Displaced Sleep on Testosterone," *Journal of Clinical Endocrinology and Metabolism* 90, no. 8 (August 2005): 4530–5, https://www.ncbi.nlm.nih.gov/pubmed/15914523.

Chapter 6

1. Donovitz, *Age Healthier, Live Happier*, 17.
2. Donovitz, *Age Healthier, Live Happier*, 33.
3. Arthritis Foundation, *Arthritis by the Numbers: Book of Trusted Facts and Figures* (2018), https://www.arthritis.org/Documents/Sections/About-Arthritis/arthritis-facts-stats-figures.pdf.
4. G. S. Lynch, "Emerging Drugs for Sarcopenia: Age-Related Muscle Wasting," *Expert Opinion on Emerging Drugs* 9, no. 2 (November 2004): 345–61, https://www.ncbi.nlm.nih.gov/pubmed/15571490.
5. E. Leifke et al., "Age-Related Changes of Serum Sex Hormones, Insulin-Like Growth Factor-1 and Sex-Hormone Binding Globulin Levels in Men: Cross-Sectional Data From a Healthy Male Cohort," *Clinical Endocrinology (Oxford)* 53, no. 6 (December 2000): 689–95.
6. G. B. Forbes, "Longitudinal Changes in Adult Fat-Free Mass: Influence of Body Weight," *American Journal of Clinical Nutrition* 70 (1999): 1025–31.
7. "Deaths and Mortality," Centers for Disease Control and Prevention, accessed September 27, 2018, https://www.cdc.gov/nchs/fastats/deaths.htm.
8. Will Brink, "Preventing Sarcopenia," *Life Extension*, January 2007, http://www.lifeextension.com/Magazine/2007/1/report_muscle/Page-01?p=1.
9. "A Profile of Older Americans 2010," Administration on Aging, September 28, 2011, https://www.acl.gov/aging-and-disability-in-america/data-and-research/profile-older-americans.
10. D. D. Thompson, "Aging and Sarcopenia," *Journal of Musculoskeletal & Neuronal Interactions* 7, no. 4 (2007): 344–5.
11. S. von Haehling, J. E. Morley, and S. D. Anker, "An Overview of Sarcopenia: Facts and Numbers on Prevalence and Clinical Impact,"

Journal of Cachexia, Sarcopenia and Muscle 1, no. 2 (December 2010): 129–33, https://www.ncbi.nlm.nih.gov/pmc/articles/PMC3060646/.

12. I. Janssen et al., "The Healthcare Costs of Sarcopenia in the United States," *Journal of the American Geriatrics Society* 52, no. 1 (January 2004): 80–85.

13. Janssen et al., "Low Relative Skeletal Muscle Mass (Sarcopenia) in Older Persons Is Associated With Functional Impairment and Physical Disability," *Journal of the American Geriatrics Society* 50, no. 5 (May 2002): 889–96.

14. Lynch, *Sarcopenia—Age-Related Muscle Wasting and Weakness.*

15. Janssen et al., "The Healthcare Costs of Sarcopenia in the United States."

16. Marcell, "Sarcopenia: Causes, Consequences, and Preventions," *Journals of Gerontology* 58 (2003): M911-M916.

17. Alliance for Aging Research, *The Silver Book: Chronic Disease and Medical Innovation in an Aging Nation*, http://silverbook.org/fact /31 29 September 2011.

18. Alliance for Aging Research, *The Silver Book.*

19. Lynch, *Sarcopenia—Age-Related Muscle Wasting and Weakness*, 334.

20. "1 in 3 Americans Will Have Diabetes by 2050, CDC Says," *Live Science*, October 22, 2010, https://www.livescience.com/10195-1-3 -americans-diabetes-2050-cdc.html.

21. "1 in 3 Americans Will Have Diabetes by 2050, CDC Says," *Live Science.*

22. Edward R. Rosick, "Protecting Muscle Mass as You Age," Life Extension, August 2003, http://www.lifeextension.com/ magazine/2003/8/report_muscle/Page-01.

23. Brink, "Preventing Sarcopenia."

24. Leifke et al., "Age-Related Changes of Serum Sex Hormones, Insulin-Like Growth Factor-1 and Sex-Hormone Binding Globulin Levels in Men."

CHAPTER 7

1. N. Asi et al., "Progesterone vs. Synthetic Progestins and the Risk of Breast Cancer: A Systematic Review and Meta-Analysis," *Systematic Reviews* 5 (2016): 121, https://www.ncbi.nlm.nih.gov/pmc/articles /PMC4960754/.

2. Edward M. Lichten, *Textbook of Bio-Identical Hormones* (Michigan: U.S. Doctors Resources LLC, 2014), 11.

3. PCCA, "Atrevis™ Hydrogel," 2017, http://files.constantcontact .com/998803f1601/89693950-dd43-47c8-ace2-d38fc86bb41d.pdf.

4. Paul J. Rosch, "America's Leading Adult Health Problem," *USA Magazine*, May 1991.

5. Intermountain Medical Center, "Testosterone Supplementation Reduces Heart Attack Risk in Men With Heart Disease,"

Science Daily, April 3, 2016, www.sciencedaily.com/
releases/2016/04/160403195920.htm.

6. P. G. Cohen, "Obesity in Men: The Hypogonadal-Estrogen Receptor
Relationship and Its Effect on Glucose Homeostasis," *Medical
Hypotheses* 70, no. 2 (2008): 358–360.

7. "Adult Obesity Facts," Centers for Disease Control and Prevention,
accessed September 27, 2018, https://www.cdc.gov/obesity
/data/adult.html.

8. "Defining Adult Overweight and Obesity," Centers for Disease Control
and Prevention, accessed September 27, 2018, https://www.cdc
.gov/obesity/adult/defining.html.

9. Pamela Smith, *HRT: The Answers* (Traverse City, MI: Healthy Living
Books Inc., 2003).

10. A. Morgentaler et al., "Prevalence of Prostate Cancer Among
Hypogonadal Men With Prostate-Specific Antigen Levels of 4.0
ng/mL or Less," *Current Therapeutic Research, Clinical and
Experimental* 68, no. 6 (December 2006): 1263-7.

11. Abraham Morgentaler, "Destroying the Myth About Testosterone
Replacement and Prostate Cancer," *Life Extension,* December 2008,
http://www.lef.org/magazine/2008/12/destroying-the-myth-about-
testosterone-replacement-prostate-cancer/page-01.

12. A. Morgentaler, "Testosterone Replacement Therapy and Prostate
Risks: Where's the Beef?," *Canadian Journal of Urology* 13,
no. 1 (February 2006): 40-3, https://www.ncbi.nlm.nih.gov/
pubmed/16526980.

13. American Thyroid Association, "Thyroid and Cholesterol," *Clinical
Thyroidology for the Public* 5, no. 12 (October 2012): 3, https://www.
thyroid.org/patient-thyroid-information/ct-for-patients/vol-5
-issue-12/p-3/.

14. Mark Starr, *Hypothyroidism Type 2* (Missouri: Mark Starr Trust,
2005), 37.

15. "Low Testosterone," American Diabetes Association, accessed
September 27, 2018, http://www.diabetes.org/living-with-diabetes
/treatment-and-care/men/low-testosterone.html.

16. R. T. Joffe, "Hormone Treatment of Depression," *Dialogues in Clinical
Neuroscience* 13, no. 1 (March 2011): 127–38, https://www.ncbi
.nlm.nih.gov/pmc/articles/PMC3181966/.

CHAPTER 8

1. Pamela Wartian Smith, *What You Must Know About Thyroid
Disorders and What to Do About Them* (New York: Square One
Publishers, 2016), 17.

2. Starr, *Hypothyroidism Type 2,* 1.

3. Broda O. Barnes, *Hypothyroidism: The Unsuspected Illness* (New
York: Harper and Row, 1939).

4. Donovitz, *Age Healthier, Live Happier,* 57.

5. Broda, *Hypothyroidism*.
6. Starr, *Hypothyroidism Type 2*, 147.
7. Starr, *Hypothyroidism Type 2*, 43.
8. Broda O. Barnes and Charlotte W. Barnes, *Hope for Hypoglycemia*, rev. ed. (American Book Company, 1999).
9. Starr, *Hypothyroidism Type 2*, 84.
10. Starr, *Hypothyroidism Type 2*, 186.
11. Cohen, *Thyroid Healthy*, 5.
12. Bowthorpe, *Stop the Thyroid Madness*, 168.
13. R. Rising et al., "Concomitant Interindividual Variation in Body Temperature and Metabolic Rate," *American Journal of Physiology* 263, no. 4 (October 1, 1992): E730–4, https://doi.org/10.1152/ajpendo.1992.263.4.E730.
14. Lichten, *Textbook of Bio-Identical Hormones*, 11.
15. A. Carle et al., "Epidemiology of Subtypes of Hypothyroidism in Denmark," *European Journal of Endocrinology* 154, no. 1 (January 2006): 21–8, https://doi.org/10.1530/eje.1.02068.
16. Lichten, *Textbook of Bio-Identical Hormones*, 63.
17. Smith, *What You Must Know About Thyroid Disorders and What to Do About Them*, 25–6.
18. Bowthorpe, *Stop the Thyroid Madness*, 50.
19. J. R. Garber et al., "Clinical Practice Guidelines for Hypothyroidism in Adults: Cosponsored by the American Association of Clinical Endocrinologists and the American Thyroid Association," *Endocrine Practice* 18, no. 6 (2012): 988–1028.
20. Starr, *Hypothyroidism Type 2*, 70.
21. Janie A. Bowthorpe, *Stop the Thyroid Madness II* (Colorado: Laughing Grape Publishing, 2014), 83.
22. "Iodine Deficiency," American Thyroid Association, accessed September 27, 2018, https://www.thyroid.org/iodine-deficiency/.
23. Katie Mui, "Why Synthroid Is the Most Prescribed Drug in the US," GoodRx, November 7, 2017, https://www.goodrx.com/blog/why-synthroid-is-the-most-prescribed-drug-in-the-us/.
24. Yusuf "JP" Saleeby, in Bowthorpe, *Stop the Thyroid Madness II*, 65.
25. Saleeby in Bowthorpe, *Stop the Thyroid Madness II*.
26. Bowthorpe, *Stop the Thyroid Madness*, 33.
27. Bowthorpe, *Stop the Thyroid Madness II*, 246.

CHAPTER 9

1. C. Steffensen et al., "Epidemiology of Cushing's Syndrome," *Neuroendocrinology* 92, no. 1 (2010): 1–5, https://doi.org/10.1159/000314297.
2. A. R. Genazzani et al., "Long-Term Low-Dose Dehydroepiandrosterone Replacement Therapy in Aging Males With Partial Androgen Deficiency," *Aging Male* 7, no. 2 (June 2004): 133–43, https://www.ncbi.nlm.nih.gov/pubmed/15672938.

3. Rosch, "America's Leading Adult Health Problem."

Chapter 10

1. Kathy C. Maupin, *The Secret Female Hormone* (Carlsbad, CA: Hay House, 2014), https://books.google.com/books?id=t0BQAwAAQBAJ&pg.
2. Brink, "Preventing Sarcopenia."
3. Maupin, *The Secret Female Hormone*, xxi.
4. Maupin, *The Secret Female Hormone*, 94.
5. Morgentaler, *Testosterone for Life*, 1.
6. Maupin, *The Secret Female Hormone*, 7.
7. Morgentaler, *Testosterone for Life*, 14.
8. R. Glaser and C. Dimitrakakis, "Testosterone Therapy in Women: Myths and Misconceptions," *Maturitas* 74, no. 3 (March 2013): 230-4, https://doi.org/10.1016/j.maturitas.2013.01.003; Maupin, *The Secret Female Hormone*, 196.
9. Maupin, *The Secret Female Hormone*, 32.
10. Maupin, *The Secret Female Hormone*, 94.
11. R. L. Cunningham et al., "Oxidative Stress, Testosterone, and Cognition Among Caucasian and Mexican American Men With and Without Alzheimer's Disease," *Journal of Alzheimer's Disease* 40, no. 3 (2014): 563–73, https://doi.org/10.3233/JAD-131994.
12. Maupin, *The Secret Female Hormone*, 94, 172.
13. Maupin, *The Secret Female Hormone*.
14. Amanda Brimhall, "Busting the Myth of Testosterone Therapy," Forever Health, February 10, 2017, https://www.foreverhealth.com/blogs/forever-health/busting-the-myth-of-testosterone-therapy.
15. M. F. Sowers et al., "Testosterone Concentrations in Women Aged 25–50 Years: Associations With Lifestyle, Body Composition, and Ovarian Status," *American Journal of Epidemiology* 153, no. 3 (February 1, 2001): 256–64, https://doi.org/10.1093/aje/153.3.256.

Chapter 11

1. Donovitz, *Age Healthier, Live Happier*, 75.
2. William Faloon, "As We See It: Surprise Findings in Estrogen Debate," *Life Extension*, November 2013, http://www.lifeextension.com/magazine/2013/11/surprise-findings-in-estrogen-debate/page-04?p=1.
3. B. Formby and T. S. Wiley, "Progesterone Inhibits Growth and Induces Apoptosis in Breast Cancer Cells: Inverse Effects on Bcl-2 and p53," *Annals of Clinical and Laboratory Science* 28, no. 6 (November–December 1998): 360–9, https://www.ncbi.nlm.nih.gov/pubmed/9846203.
4. J. E. Rossouw et al., "Risks and Benefits of Estrogen Plus Progestin in Healthy Postmenopausal Women: Principal Results From the Women's Health Initiative Randomized Controlled Trial," *JAMA*

288, no. 3 (July 2002): 321–33, https://www.ncbi.nlm.nih.gov/pubmed/12117397; Y. Liang et al., "Synthetic Progestins Induce Growth and Metastasis of BT-474 Human Breast Cancer Xenografts in Nude Mice," *Menopause* 17, no. 5 (September–October 2010): 1040–7, https://doi.org/10.1097/gme.0b013e3181d3dd0c; J. V. Porch et al., "Estrogen-Progestin Replacement Therapy and Breast Cancer Risk: The Women's Health Study (United States)," *Cancer Causes and Control* 13, no. 9 (November 2002): 847–54, https://www.ncbi.nlm.nih.gov/pubmed/12462550.

5. G. Plu-Bureau et al., "Percutaneous Progesterone Use and Risk of Breast Cancer: Results From a French Cohort Study of Premenopausal Women With Benign Breast Disease," *Cancer Detection and Prevention* 23, no. 4 (1999): 290–6, https://www.ncbi.nlm.nih.gov/pubmed/10403900.

6. U. Larsson-Cohn et al., "Lipoprotein Changes May Be Minimized by Proper Composition of a Combined Oral Contraceptive," *Fertility and Sterility* 35, no. 2 (February 1981): 172–9, https://www.ncbi.nlm.nih.gov/pubmed/7193603.

7. Melissa Conrad Stoppler, "Menopause (Symptoms, Remedies, and Treatment Medications)," WebMD Inc., accessed October 1, 2018, https://www.emedicinehealth.com/menopause/article_em.htm #definition_and_facts_about_menopause.

8. "Progesterone," Laboratory Corporation of America Holdings, accessed August 21, 2018, https://www.labcorp.com/test-menu/33596 /progesterone.

CHAPTER 12

1. Maupin, *The Secret Female Hormone*, 172.

2. Lichten, *Textbook of Bio-Identical Hormones*, 117.

3. K. M. Webber, "The Contribution of Luteinizing Hormone to Alzheimer Disease Pathogenesis," *Clinical Medicine and Research* 5, no. 3 (October 2007): 177¬–83, https://doi.org/10.3121/cmr.2007.741.

4. Maupin, *The Secret Female Hormone*, 125.

5. N. J. Raine-Fenning, M. P. Brincat, and Y. Muscat-Baron, "Skin Aging and Menopause: Implications for Treatment," *American Journal of Clinical Dermatology* 4, no. 6 (February 2003): 371-8, https://www.ncbi.nlm.nih.gov/pubmed/12762829.

6. M. A. Kirschner et al., "Obesity, Hormones, and Cancer," *Cancer Research* 41, no. 9 (September 1981): 3711–7, https://www.ncbi.nlm.nih.gov/pubmed/7260928.

7. Pamela Smith, *What You Must Know About Women's Hormones* (Garden City Park, NY: Square One Publishers, 2010), 17; Amy Lee Hawkins, *What You Must Know About Bioidentical Hormone Replacement Therapy* (New York: Square One Publishing, 2013), 89.

CHAPTER 13

1. A. Colmou, "Estrogens and Vascular Thrombosi," *Soins. Gynécologie, Obstétrique, Puériculture, Pédiatrie* 16 (September 1982): 39–41, https://www.ncbi.nlm.nih.gov/pubmed/6925385.
2. R. D. Abbott et al., "Serum Estradiol and Risk of Stroke in Elderly Men," *Neurology* 68, no. 8 (February 20, 2007): 563–8.
3. G. Carruba, "Estrogen and Prostate Cancer: An Eclipsed Truth in an Androgen-Dominated Scenario," *Journal of Cellular Biochemistry* 102, no. 4 (November 1, 2007): 899–911, https://doi.org/10.1002/jcb.21529; J. L. Nelles, W. Hu, and G. S. Prins, "Estrogen Action and Prostate Cancer," *Expert Review of Endocrinology & Metabolism* 6, no. 3 (May 2011): 437–51, https://doi.org/10.1586/eem.11.20.
4. E. L. Klaiber et al., "Serum Estrogen Levels in Men With Acute Myocardial Infarction," *American Journal of Medicine* 73, no. 6 (December 1982): 872–81, https://www.ncbi.nlm.nih.gov/pubmed/7148879; G. B. Phillips, B. H. Pinkernell, and T. Jing, "The Association of Hyperestrogenemia With Coronary Thrombosis in Men," *Arteriosclerosis, Thrombosis, and Vascular Biology* 16 (2018): 1383–7, https://doi.org/10.1161/atvb.16.11.1383.

CHAPTER 14

1. Campbell and Brown, *The Testosterone Optimization Therapy Bible,* 12; T. G. Travison et al., "A Population-Level Decline in Serum Testosterone Levels in American Men," *Journal of Clinical Endocrinology and Metabolism* 92, no. 1 (January 2007): 196–202, https://doi.org/10.1210/jc.2006-1375.
2. Jay Campbell, *The Definitive Testosterone Replacement Therapy Manual* (Archangel Ink, 2015), 39.
3. D. A. Gruenewald and A. M. Matsumoto, "Testosterone Supplementation Therapy for Older Men: Potential Benefits and Risks," *Journal of the American Geriatrics Society* 51, no. 1 (January 2003): 101–15, https://www.ncbi.nlm.nih.gov/pubmed/12534854.
4. P. G. Cohen, "Obesity in Men: The Hypogonadal—Estrogen Receptor Relationship and Its Effect on Glucose Homeostasis," *Medical Hypotheses* 70, no. 2 (2008): 358–60.
5. L. H. Goh, C. H. How, and T. C. Lau, "Male Osteoporosis: Clinical Approach and Management in Family Practice," *Singapore Medical Journal* 55, no. 7 (July 2014): 353–7, https://www.ncbi.nlm.nih.gov/pubmed/25091882.
6. H. A. Fink et al., "Association of Testosterone and Estradiol Deficiency With Osteoporosis and Rapid Bone Loss in Older Men," *Journal of Clinical Endocrinology and Metabolism* 91, no. 10 (October 2006): 3908–15, https://doi.org/10.1210/jc.2006-0173.
7. R. L. Cunningham et al., "Oxidative Stress, Testosterone, and Cognition Among Caucasian and Mexican American Men With and

Without Alzheimer's Disease," *Journal of Alzheimer's Disease* 40, no. 3 (2014): 563–73, https://doi.org/10.3233/JAD-131994.

8. A. D. Mooradian, J. E. Morley, and S. G. Korenman, "Biological Actions of Androgens," *Endocrine Reviews* 8, no. 1 (February 1987): 1–28, https://doi.org/10.1210/edrv-8-1-1.

9. C. Huggins and C. V. Hodges, "Studies on Prostatic Cancer. I. The Effect of Castration, of Estrogen and Androgen Injection on Serum Phosphatases in Metastatic Carcinoma of the Prostate," *CA: A Cancer Journal for Clinicians* 22, no. 4 (July–August 1972): 232–40, http://cancerres.aacrjournals.org/content/1/4/293?iss=4.

10. Morgentaler, *Testosterone for Life*, 135.

11. N. E. Eaton et al., "Endogenous Sex Hormones and Prostate Cancer: A Quantitative Review of Prospective Studies," *British Journal of Cancer* 80, no. 7 (June 1999): 930–34, https://doi.org/10.1038/sj.bjc.6690445.

12. Endogenous Hormones and Prostate Cancer Collaborative Group, "Endogenous Sex Hormones and Prostate Cancer: A Collaborative Analysis of 18 Prospective Studies," *Journal of the National Cancer Institute* 100, no. 3 (February 6, 2008): 170–83, https://doi.org/10.1093/jnci/djm323.

13. Morgentaler, *Testosterone for Life*, 132.

14. A. D. Mooradian, J. E. Morley, and S. G. Korenman, "Biological Actions of Androgens," 1–28.

15. C. Ohlsson et al., "High Serum Testosterone Is Associated With Reduced Risk of Cardiovascular Events in Elderly Men. The MrOS (Osteoporotic Fractures in Men) Study in Sweden," *Journal of the American College of Cardiology* 58, no. 16 (October 11, 2011): 1674–81, https://doi.org/10.1016/j.jacc.2011.07.019.

16. B. Gencer and F. Mach, "Testosterone: A Hormone Preventing Cardiovascular Disease or a Therapy Increasing Cardiovascular Events?," *European Heart Journal* 37, no. 48 (December 21, 2016): 3569–75, https://doi.org/10.1093/eurheartj/ehv439.

17. J. Baillargeon et al., "Risk of Venous Thromboembolism in Men Receiving Testosterone Therapy," *Mayo Clinic Proceedings* 90, no. 8 (August 2015): 1038–1045, https://doi.org/10.1016/j.mayocp.2015.05.012.

18. "Educational Commentary—Testosterone and Sex-Hormone Binding Globulin," American Proficiency Institute, accessed September 27, 2018, http://www.api-pt.com/Reference/Commentary/2013Achem.pdf.

19. Ohlsson et al., "High Serum Testosterone Is Associated With Reduced Risk of Cardiovascular Events in Elderly Men."

20. Donovitz, *Age Healthier, Live Happier*, 83.

21. Juan Augustine Galindo Jr., "Normal Estradiol Levels in Men," Testosterone Centers of Texas, September 27, 2016, https://tctmed.com/normal-estradiol-levels/.

22. "Educational Commentary—Testosterone and Sex-Hormone Binding Globulin," American Proficiency Institute.

23. K. M. Lakshman et al., "The Effects of Injected Testosterone Dose and Age on the Conversion of Testosterone to Estradiol and Dihydrotestosterone in Young and Older Men," *Journal of Clinical Endocrinology and Metabolism* 95, no. 8 (August 2010): 3955–64, https://doi.org/10.1210/jc.2010-0102.

24. Amanda Brimhall, "Busting the Myth of Testosterone Therapy," Forever Health, February 10, 2017, https://www.foreverhealth .com/blogs/forever-health/busting-the-myth-of-testosterone-therapy.

25. "A Population-Level Decline in Serum Testosterone Levels in American Men," *Journal of Clinical Endocrinology and Metabolism* 92, no. 1 (January 2007): 196–202, https://doi.org/10.1210/jc.2006-1375.

26. P. G. Cohen. "Aromatase, Adiposity, Aging and Disease. The Hypogonadal-Metabolic-Atherogenic-Disease and Aging Connection," *Medical Hypotheses* 56, no. 6 (June 2001): 702-8, https://doi. org/10.1054/mehy.2000.1169; P. G. Cohen, "The Hypogonadal-Obesity Cycle: Role of Aromatase in Modulating the Testosterone-Estradiol Shunt—a Major Factor in the Genesis of Morbid Obesity," *Medical Hypotheses* 52, no. 1 (January 1999): 49–51, https://doi.org/10.1054/ mehy.1997.0624.

CHAPTER 15

1. G. E. Butterfield, "The Effects of Recombinant Human Insulin-Like Growth Factor-1 and Growth Hormone on Body Composition in Elderly Women," *Journal of Clinical Endocrinology and Metabolism* 80, no. 6 (June 1995): 1845–52, https://doi.org/10.1210/ jcem.80.6.7539817.

2. D. Rudman et al., "Effects of Human Growth Hormone in Men Over 60 Years Old," *New England Journal of Medicine* 323, no. 1 (July 5, 1990): 1–6, https://doi.org/10.1056/NEJM199007053230101.

3. R. R. Suminski et al., "Acute Effect of Amino Acid Ingestion and Resistance Exercise on Plasma Growth Hormone Concentration in Young Men," *International Journal of Sport Nutrition* 7, no. 1 (March 1997): 48–60, https://www.ncbi.nlm.nih.gov/pubmed/9063764.

4. T. C. Welbourne, "Increased Plasma Bicarbonate and Growth Hormone After an Oral Glutamine Load," *American Journal of Clinical Nutrition* 61, no. 5 (May 1995): 1058–61, https://www.ncbi. nlm.nih.gov/pubmed/7733028.

APPENDIX D

1. Bowthorpe, *Stop the Thyroid Madness II*, 217.

2. Cohen, *Thyroid Healthy*, 89.

3. Bowthorpe, *Stop the Thyroid Madness II*, 190.

APPENDIX G

1. "12 Worst Endocrine Disruptors Revealed by Environmental Working
   Group and Keep a Breast," Keep a Breast, October 29, 2013, http://
   keep-a-breast.org/12-worst-endocrine-disruptors-revealed
   -environment/; "Dirty Dozen Endocrine Disruptors: 12 Hormone
   -Altering Chemicals and How to Avoid Them," Environmental
   Working Group, October 28, 2013, https://www.ewg.org/research/
   dirty-dozen-list-endocrine-disruptors#.W23oQtJKgb4.

INDEX

F

facial hair 28, 128, 149

fatigue xiii–xiv, 5, 14, 16, 27–28, 39, 57, 63, 70, 85–87, 89–90, 97–98, 106–107, 109–116, 118–120, 122, 126, 139, 157, 170, 174, 187, 195, 208

ferritin 43, 208

fibromyalgia xv, 5, 28, 54, 66, 76, 98, 109, 111, 120, 139–140, 191, 195

fingernails 28, 30, 87, 90, 97, 158, 186

fluid retention 28, 90, 112, 141, 191

fluoride 43, 96

focus ix, 4, 7, 52, 71, 81, 89, 112, 158, 170, 175

follicle-stimulating hormone. *See* FSH

forgiveness 38, 117–118, 140, 195, 202

frailty xv, 21, 28, 54–55, 60, 167, 169, 187

FSH 61, 123, 151–157, 159, 205, 214

G

gallstones 13, 159

gels 22, 72–73, 162, 179–180, 183

glaucoma 195

glutamine 189, 193

glutathione 37, 207, 212

gluten 37, 75, 100, 124, 147, 208

gynecomastia 12, 29, 42, 45, 164, 172, 182

H

hair loss xv, 15–16, 27, 29, 43, 86, 90, 97, 112, 127, 142, 159, 180, 182

Hashimoto's thyroiditis 35–37, 43, 75, 89, 91, 94, 178, 195, 208

headaches 14, 112, 124, 141, 149, 191

heart attacks 13, 17–23, 77, 93, 132, 134, 143, 157, 174, 182

heart disease xiii–xiv, 13, 17–18, 20, 23–24, 29, 31, 40, 45, 52, 58, 60, 66, 77, 88, 90, 99, 110, 112, 115, 126, 162, 164, 170, 173, 177–178, 183, 188, 195, 211, 215

heart rate. *See* pulse

HGH 65, 185 187, 189 193, 207

high blood pressure xiii–xiv, 5, 13, 22, 29, 45, 89–90, 106, 109–110, 115, 168

hormone disruptors 37–45, 55, 82, 86, 88, 96, 125, 127, 163, 171, 183, 209, 215–216

hormone replacement therapy 6, 10–12, 16–19, 23, 25–26, 32, 50, 55, 58, 65, 69–71, 73–74, 76–78, 82, 125, 152, 156, 161–162, 169, 171, 178, 195

hot flashes 14, 76, 123, 127, 152

human growth hormone. *See* HGH

hydrocortisone 120–122, 140

hypertension. *See* high blood pressure

hyperthyroidism 35, 89, 93, 95

hypothalamus 86

hypothyroidism 35–36, 43, 88–94, 97–98, 101, 108, 130. *See also* thyroid hormones

hysterectomy 44, 54, 123–124, 143–145, 159

I

IBS 29, 116, 208

IGF-1 187–190, 192, 194

immune system 35, 81, 106, 121, 134, 137, 186, 203

infertility xv, 29, 38, 40, 88, 90, 112, 144, 215–216

inflammation xv, 53, 57, 59, 63, 65, 80, 109, 111, 121, 133, 167, 169, 204, 208

injections 4, 20, 67, 72–73, 87, 135, 155–156, 159, 161–162, 165, 168, 179–180, 183, 185, 189–190, 193

insomnia xiii, 5, 7, 10, 14, 19, 29, 45, 76, 90, 110–113, 119, 126 127, 139, 141, 145, 170, 175, 195

insulin 29, 40, 80, 90, 157, 188, 207

    insulin resistance 45, 62–63, 66, 80–81

    insulin tolerance test 187–188, 193

insulin-like growth factor 1. *See* IGF-1

iodine 36–37, 43, 95, 119, 201, 207, 211, 216

iron 43, 119, 208, 212

irritability 3, 5, 16, 19, 29, 44, 49, 60, 90, 97, 112, 122–123, 125–126, 128–129, 134, 140–141, 143–144, 149, 167, 170, 175

FREE Resources for you

Thank you for reading my book. In today's society, it's so important to understand the technologies and tests that are available to you, whether you want to feel 25 again, or if you are experiencing symptoms that doctors haven't been able to explain.

I encourage you to explore beyond what is presented in this book. So as a **THANK YOU** and a way for you to take action, I am offering you a couple of resources to take with you to your next visit with your doctor:

FREE Pamphlet:

Optimize Your Body, Optimize Your Life!
(Record your symptoms, get blood tests, and compare results using this reference pamphlet)

FREE Infographic:

Add These Tests to My Blood Panel
(A quick guide on which hormone tests to ask for on your next blood panel)

To get these **FREE** gifts, please visit:
HormoneHealthBook.com/gift

Blessings,

Dr. Don Colbert

16106